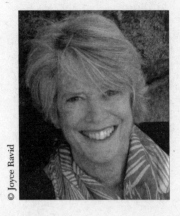

© Joyce Ravid

KATHERINE BOUTON is a former editor at *The New York Times,* where she worked for *The New York Times Magazine* and *The New York Times Book Review,* as well as the daily Science and Culture desks. Her nonfiction has appeared in *The New Yorker, The New York Times Magazine,* and many other magazines and reviews, and she is a regular reviewer and contributor to Tuesday's Science Times section. She is a member of the Board of Trustees of the Hearing Loss Association of America. She lives in New York City with her husband, Daniel Menaker. They have two grown children.

SHOUTING WON'T HELP

SHOUTING WON'T HELP

Why I—and 50 Million Other Americans—Can't Hear You

Katherine Bouton

Picador

———

A Sarah Crichton Book
Farrar, Straus and Giroux
New York

SHOUTING WON'T HELP. Copyright © 2013 by Katherine Bouton.
Introduction copyright © 2014 by Katherine Bouton. All rights reserved.
Printed in the United States of America. For information, address
Picador, 175 Fifth Avenue, New York, N.Y. 10010.

www.picadorusa.com
www.twitter.com/picadorusa • www.facebook.com/picadorusa
picadorbookroom.tumblr.com

Picador® is a U.S. registered trademark and is used by Farrar,
Straus and Giroux under license from Pan Books Limited.

For book club information, please visit www.facebook.com/picadorbookclub
or e-mail marketing@picadorusa.com.

Designed by Jonathan D. Lippincott

The Library of Congress has cataloged the Farrar, Straus and Giroux edition as follows:

Bouton, Katherine, 1947–
    Shouting won't help: why I—and 50 million other Americans—
can't hear you / Katherine Bouton.
        p. cm.
    Includes bibliographical references and index.
    ISBN 978-0-374-26304-1 (hardcover)
    ISBN 978-1-4299-5337-5 (e-book)
    1. Bouton, Katherine, 1947– 2. Deaf women—New York (State)—
New York—Biography. 3. Deafness. I. Title.
RF290 B58 2013
617.8092—dc23
[B]

                                                    2012029096

Picador ISBN 978-1-250-04356-6

Picador books may be purchased for educational, business, or promotional use.
For information on bulk purchases, please contact Macmillan Corporate and
Premium Sales Department at 1-800-221-7945, extension 5442, or write
specialmarkets@macmillan.com.

First published in the United States by Sarah Crichton Books,
an imprint of Farrar, Straus and Giroux

First Picador Edition: February 2014

10 9 8 7 6 5 4 3 2 1

For Dan

Contents

SHOUTING WON'T HELP

Introduction to the 2014 Edition

How many people do you know who are deaf? Not stone-deaf, but not able to hear much either. How many do you know who say "What?" too often, who seem uncharacteristically befuddled or aloof, who don't go to parties anymore? Not Deaf, with a capital *D*. Just deaf. Deaf like me.

When I was thirty, one minute I could hear and the next I couldn't. My left ear went dead. Eventually, I regained some of the hearing, but not all. I was young, and I ignored it (just as I ignored the recommendation for a hearing aid). It never occurred to me that this was the first step toward a far more serious impairment. In the years that followed, I would experience other random assaults on my hearing, and by the time I was forty my hearing loss was serious enough to affect my daily life. By fifty, I was losing the hearing in the other ear as well, and wore hearing aids in both ears. By sixty, I was functionally deaf.

I have sensorineural hearing loss, the kind that affects the majority of people with hearing loss. It is usually caused by a defect in the hair cells of the inner ear. What caused the defect in *my* hair cells remains a mystery, as it does for 75 percent of people who experience sudden hearing loss. I do hear, thanks to a cochlear implant in my left ear—surgically embedded in my skull—and a powerful hearing aid in my right. But like many people with severe hearing loss, my hearing cannot be fully corrected. Even with both devices, I say "What?" so often that my husband has asked me to occasionally substitute "Pardon me?" or "Huh?" I like "Sorry?"

People with moderate to severe loss can't hear if they can't see the speaker face to face. They can't hear in a group. They can't hear in an airport terminal or on a noisy street. I can't either. But without my devices I also can't hear an alarm clock, a fire alarm, the telephone ringing, the vacuum cleaner, a siren. I can sleep through a violent thunderstorm. I've been known to sleep through my iPhone alarm, my "Shake-n-Wake" vibrating alarm clock, and a hotel wake-up call—all on the same morning.

Chances are you know quite a few people who have trouble hearing. But you probably don't always know who they are. Hearing loss is one of America's best-kept secrets. People don't want to acknowledge hearing loss. They fear that it's a sign of aging.

Because hearing loss is a hidden disability, it's very hard to state how many people it affects. The National Institute on Deafness and Other Communication Disorders (NIDCD) states that 36 million people, or 17 percent of the population, report some degree of hearing loss. (On the face of it, this figure makes no sense. The 2013 population is 315 million—17 percent of that is 53 million.) Yet, in 2011, Frank Lin and colleagues at Johns Hopkins published a well-regarded study establishing that 48 million have some degree of loss. How can such a basic piece of information—the number of people with hearing loss—vary so widely?

Lin's study used audiometric tests to assess whether a participant had hearing loss. The NIDCD bases its number on self-report, a method that is not likely to provide an accurate figure: many people don't acknowledge hearing loss even to themselves. Most hearing loss organizations, including the Hearing Health Foundation, now accept Frank Lin's figure of 48 million as the most accurate.

But however you count it, nearly one in five people, across all age groups, has trouble understanding speech, and many cannot hear certain sounds at all.

. . .

When I first learned how many Americans had hearing loss, I was astounded. Tens of millions more people with hearing problems than vision problems? Why don't we know this? Once again, the explanation is the association of hearing loss with aging.

The older you are, it's true, the more likely you'll have hearing loss. But—and this can be hard to get your mind around—more than half the people in America with hearing loss are under the age of fifty-five. Among American males with hearing loss, the NIDCD tells us, 32 percent began to lose their hearing between the ages of twenty and thirty-nine, and another 32 percent between forty and fifty-nine. Sixty-four percent of American males with hearing loss, that is, began to lose their hearing before they were sixty. Hearing loss affects every age group, including adolescents. A 2010 study found that 19.5 percent of teens have at least slight hearing loss, and 5 percent have hearing loss so serious they can't hear a whisper. Your teenager may not be ignoring you but truly may not hear you.

Those numbers should dispel the myth that hearing loss is a condition of aging. Unfortunately, they don't. And here's why:

Hearing loss may not be a condition of aging, but it *is* a condition of the elderly. Two-thirds of Americans seventy and older have a hearing impairment. But in only 8 percent of men and 16 percent of women did the loss begin after the age of seventy. The vast majority had started to lose their hearing decades earlier. Since many younger people are loathe to admit the loss, the result is the misperception that people with hearing loss are elderly.

The overall number of people with hearing loss should have gone down, rather than up. We have eliminated most of the childhood diseases, like meningitis, scarlet fever, mumps, and measles, that can cause hearing loss. Our society has moved from a noisy industrial manufacturing base to a postindustrial service- and information-based economy. OSHA regulates noise exposure in the workplace. We are healthier than ever. Life expectancy keeps going up.

Worldwide, 380 million people have "disabling" hearing loss, according to a 2013 report by the World Health Organization. The economic impact is enormous: "In developing countries, children with hearing loss and deafness rarely receive any schooling," the report states. "Adults with hearing loss also have a much higher unemployment rate."

• • •

Not only can it be hard to admit to hearing loss, but because the onset is usually gradual, it's also sometimes unrecognized. Friends and family may point out that a loved one seems to be having trouble hearing, only to be met with excuses. "I can hear just fine . . . People talk too fast . . . It's too noisy in this restaurant . . . at this party . . . on this bus. The phone isn't working properly . . . My wife mumbles."

Only one in five people who could benefit from a hearing aid uses one, according to the NIDCD. But just as people deny hearing loss, they overstate hearing aid use. They may own hearing aids, but keep them in a drawer. Frank Lin also studied hearing aid use, again using audiometric testing. He found that only one in *seven* over the age of fifty who could benefit used hearing aids. (For working-age adults fifty to fifty-nine, the number drops to one in twenty.) In developing countries, according to WHO, the number is one in forty. The average lapse between the time a doctor recommends hearing aids and the time the user actually gets them is seven years. Many wait decades. I did.

But you ignore hearing loss at your peril, and not only from the depression and isolation that accompanies untreated hearing loss. As I realized when I got a cochlear implant, it had been so many years since I'd heard anything out of that left ear that I had, in essence, forgotten how to. The speech pathways in my brain had altered to a point where rebooting them was very difficult.

Some cite cost as a factor in the low use of hearing aids. A standard quality hearing aid costs between $2000 and $6000. In the

United States, the expense has until now not been covered by private health insurance, Medicare, or Medicaid. (Some insurers are beginning to cover a portion of the cost of certain kinds of hearing aids. Twenty states mandate some form of coverage for hearing aids for children.) But as numbers in the U.K. show, the stigma of aging plays a role in this as well. Hearing aids are free under the National Health Service, but only one in three citizens who needs a hearing aid has one.

A further deterrent—and something the hearing aid companies would rather you didn't know—is that they often don't work very well, especially for those with severe loss. The human ear is a miraculous thing, allowing us to hear a multitude of subtle differences in sound, to screen out background noise, to shut down when things get loud. A hearing aid or implant does all these things, but poorly. Neither is a substitute for the real thing.

. . .

When I started my research for this book, I had been struggling with increasingly severe hearing loss for much of a decade. I was depressed, anxious, angry, stalled in my work, isolated from my family and friends. After the hardcover edition of this book was published, I got e-mails day after day from people thanking me for describing what their life was like. "Your own personal pain, anger, sadness, exhaustion, and isolation are all a part of my world, too," one man wrote, echoing others.

In writing this book, I thought it was important to be honest. Hearing loss is not easy. It affects friendships, family, and professional relationships. For many of us, it is a constant in our daily activities. It affects everything from a simple exchange with a store clerk to comforting a bereaved widow. We are never sure we've heard correctly. We are never sure we've responded appropriately. That's stressful.

But acknowledging the loss, sharing the experience, and finding others who have hearing loss can help mitigate this anxiety. One place to start is the Hearing Loss Association of America, the country's largest advocacy group for those with hearing loss, which has chapters in many areas. ALDA, the Association of Late-Deafened Adults, also has regional chapters. Being with others who understand your experience is a huge relief. Sometimes it's even fun. But it's also a way to get tips about dealing with hearing loss, to discover places that are accessible to the hard of hearing, venues that provide captioning or looping. It's also a way to get involved in advocacy, perhaps even to help wipe out the stigma of hearing loss.

· · ·

The structure of this book loosely follows my own progressive loss, beginning with the partial decline in my left ear at thirty, and continuing through the increasingly severe drops I experienced in subsequent years. Chapter 1 deals with the first loss, how it happened and how it affected me. As my hearing worsened, I became obsessed with finding the cause, an explanation, hoping—futilely—that I could halt the decline. In chapter 2, I discuss the causes of hearing loss. I interviewed many neuro-otologists and otolaryngologists about the causes of hearing loss, searched my own past for a clue. The researchers were generous in elucidating the mechanics of hearing and the ways it can be damaged; my past offered a hypothesis, but in the end I still had no diagnosis.

Given that the most common cause of hearing loss is noise, the more I read, the more horrified I was by the damage we are doing to ourselves. We love noise, and it's making us deaf. In chapter 3, I look at our noisy environment: from the competition in sports for the loudest stadiums to restaurants that use noise as stimulus and decor. I look at the noise in malls; the noise of games, toys, machinery; the noise of the ever-present TV not only at home but in airport lounges and doctors' offices; the noise of PA systems. Public policy has largely ignored the health issues of noise, with enormous consequences.

Ironically, the same noise that causes hearing loss also makes life even more difficult for those with hearing loss, especially if they wear hearing aids, which often can't screen it out. For many with hearing loss, noise can literally be painful.

Hearing loss has been stigmatized since prebiblical times. In chapters 4 and 5, I look at why that stigma remains pervasive today. It can be a source of anguish to the hard of hearing, yet is rarely noticed or acknowledged by others. And it keeps many from getting the treatment they need.

Hearing aids and cochlear implants, the subjects of chapters 6 through 9, have both benefits and disadvantages. Controversies and quandaries about hearing aids abound: what brand and style to buy, where to get them (online, in a big box store, or from an audiologist), how much to pay for them, how to find a good and honest audiologist, how to know if you're being ripped off.

Cochlear implants can restore hearing that seemed irretrievably lost, but they are useful to only a minority of those with hearing loss. They are most successful in children who are born deaf and who receive the implants as infants. But controversy rages here as well: shouldn't the child have a say? To wait, however, is to greatly reduce the efficacy of the implant. For adults with acquired hearing loss, the results are mixed. For some, the implant is a miracle. For me, the miracle came with reservations. Where before I had been deaf, now I could hear. But it took me several years of hard work, of formal auditory rehabilitation as well as constant use, to hear well with the implant. Now, I couldn't live without it.

Despite the Americans with Disabilities Act, hearing loss can present an insuperable obstacle in the workplace, the subject of chapter 10. For two decades I worked in a competitive environment as a senior editor at *The New York Times*. For many of those years I had a serious, unacknowledged disability. Eventually it just became too difficult and I took early retirement. At first I felt unmoored, severed from my identity, which was intricately bound to my work. In the end, leaving my job forced me to confront my hearing loss. We need a better understanding of the toll that hearing loss takes in the workplace, as well as the many technological advances that could help make the workplace more accessible.

Hearing loss rarely occurs in isolation. In chapter 11, I look at its two most common companions: tinnitus and vertigo. For those who suffer severe tinnitus or vertigo, the disorders may be harder to tolerate than hearing loss itself. And they are equally difficult to treat.

For the first time ever, a biological cure for hearing loss seems not only possible but probable. Research in gene therapy, molecular therapy, stem cell technology, and the regeneration of hair cells is advancing at a breathtaking rate. Within a decade, we may see the beginning of the end of the ravages of sensorineural hearing loss like mine.

In the meantime, prevention and protection are the best alternatives. As awareness of the dangers of noise spreads, many more people are wearing hearing protection when doing ordinary chores like mowing the lawn. The military has funded much of the research into prevention, acknowledging the impact battlefield noise has taken on its troops. Tinnitus and hearing loss are the two largest sources of disability claims among troops returning from Iraq and Afghanistan, as they were in Vietnam veterans.

• • •

Living with someone with hearing loss can try even the most patient. Hearing loss is frustrating. Those who suffer from it may dominate the conversation (it's so much easier to do all the talking yourself), they may isolate themselves, they are often angry. Not fun people to be around. These days, I acknowledge my hearing loss to longtime acquaintances as well as to people I've just met. The positive and generous responses make me wonder why I subjected myself to decades of "faking it," to the stress of pretending to be someone I wasn't.

At the end of each chapter are sections titled "Voices," short profiles of people with hearing loss, mostly in their own words.

Their backgrounds and professions differ, as do the causes and severity of their hearing loss. Some have accepted the fact of their loss, while others are still coming to terms with it. Their stories illuminate mine and cumulatively produce a portrait of the broad and devastating effect of hearing loss, as well as the peace of mind that comes with acceptance.

I learned some important things from my loss. Tolerance and understanding of what it means to suffer from a hidden disability—from serious depression or anxiety, from epilepsy, from debilitating back pain, from claustrophobia or agoraphobia, from food allergies, from alcoholism or drug addiction. Unless you've been there, it's hard to comprehend what the problem is.

It was only when I lost my hearing that I became aware of how important hearing is in establishing one's sense of place. Hearing anchors you in the world. It puts you at the center of a multidimensional universe. We hear things behind us, above us; we hear our stomachs rumble and our hearts beat. We hear in the dark; we hear in a cave or windowless cell. We hear in our sleep. Sometimes we hear in a coma. Babies hear in the womb. We hear as we breathe—effortlessly—until we can't.

Helen Keller famously said that she regarded deafness as "a much worse misfortune" than blindness, because it cuts the sufferer off from "the intellectual company of man." In the darkest days of my hearing loss, I agreed with her. But now I realize that deafness can be treated in a way not yet available to the blind. I will always be able to hear, thanks to technology.

Hearing loss continues to be an impediment, but it no longer defines me. I've stopped thinking of myself as hearing impaired, and started thinking of myself as someone with a hearing impairment.

One last thought about terminology: "Deaf" has become not just a diagnosis but a political statement. When capitalized, "Deaf" refers to a close-knit cultural community, people who use American Sign Language, or ASL. They may wear hearing aids in addition to signing, but if they choose to be part of the community, they are Deaf. They are proudly Deaf. If the child of two Deaf parents is born Deaf, quite often the parents will be relieved because the child will more naturally join their community.

Those of us with hearing loss lack not only the cohesive community of the Deaf, but a convenient term to describe ourselves. "Hearing impaired" is frowned on. "Hard of hearing" is cumbersome. One person I interviewed poignantly referred to himself as "hearing lost." Many with severe hearing loss refer to themselves as deaf, because in fact they—we—are deaf, just as a person who has lost a leg but walks with a prosthetic device is an amputee. "Deaf" used to be the default term for anyone with hearing loss. It described your great-grandmother with her hearing trumpet, or your father or grandfather with a large hearing aid that whistled and shrieked. Today the term "deaf" is politically incorrect for someone like me. But I like the word "deaf." It's blunt, sassy. It's a way to talk back to your handicap.

How to Talk to People with Hearing Loss

It can be frustrating to talk to someone who says "What?" after every sentence. Here are some tips to make the conversation easier for you both.

Shouting won't help. Speak in a normal voice and articulate as clearly as possible.

Look at the other person when you talk. Most people with hearing loss read body language and lips intuitively. Don't lean in to their ear—they need to see your lips. Look at them, not down at papers on your desk or over their heads to see who else is around.

Don't repeat yourself. If the person with hearing loss doesn't get what you said, don't simply say it again. Rephrase it. Put it into some context.

Don't give up. Once you've tried unsuccessfully two or three times, don't say, "Never mind, it doesn't matter." By the time you get to that third try, everything matters.

Consider your location. Most people with hearing loss have a difficult time in noisy places, even ones you may think are quiet. A loud air conditioner, a humming fish tank, a fan, or a TV can interfere. Turn off the background noise when they come to visit.

Make sure you have their full attention. I can't cook and hear at the same time, no matter how collegial it may seem to join me in the kitchen.

ONE

Losing It

I lost my hearing one early spring day in 1978. I was at home, writing about a trip I had made to Turkey the summer before. I had been part of an archaeological dig in southwestern Turkey, the site of a former Classical Greek and then Byzantine city. I hoped to write about the experience in a feature article for *The New Yorker*. Although I had worked at the magazine for eight years, since graduating from college, I didn't discuss the story with an editor or ask for an assignment—only for a three-month unpaid leave. I don't think a man would have been as reticent, or a young woman today. But it was 1977.

The dig was an adventure and the archaeologist in charge a vivid and controversial character. After I got home, I started writing. I was excited, happy, and slightly anxious, the way you are when you're on the brink of something that could change your life.

At some point in the morning, the phone rang and I picked it up. "Hello?" I said. "Hello????" Why couldn't I hear the caller? I tried the other ear, the right. It worked just fine.

I went over the explanations that come to anyone with sudden hearing loss. Maybe I had wax in my ear, an infection; had I forgotten some loud noise? Once before, I had lost my hearing for almost a day after being at a loud rock concert (The Who, Madison Square Garden, March 1976). It came back on its own. So would this, I thought. Or a doctor would fix it.

As the day went on, I was dizzy and my ear was crackling. Loud noises were uncomfortably amplified and startling. I went outside to clear my head, but a city bus going by whooshed its air brakes and the sound was so loud the impact felt almost physical. At home, the ring of the telephone was high-pitched and shrill; my hairbrush made a jangly clatter when I dropped it. In the evening, my soon-to-be husband, Dan, came home. He puttered around doing ordinary things—rustling paper, setting a dish on a counter, watching TV, scraping a chair on the floor. Nothing sounded like what it was, and everything sounded painfully loud.

Eventually, over the next few weeks, the crackling receded and the sensitivity stabilized. But I never regained my hearing. A doctor couldn't fix it. A doctor couldn't even figure out what had caused it. It would continue to deteriorate in fits and starts, as unexpectedly and mysteriously as that first time, with increasing frequency. Thirty years later, I was profoundly deaf in my left ear and headed in that direction in my right.

• • •

There are many things I have failed to hear, but one stands out from the others. My father died in 2010. I had been with him a lot during his illness, but I wasn't there when he went into the final stages of dying. The last words he said to me were on the phone. I didn't hear them.

My father was six foot five, 230 pounds. He wore a size 15 shoe. He'd been in the Navy in World War II and Korea, and was always trying to persuade my mother to join him on a cruise around the world—the sea was the only place big enough for him. During my childhood, he traveled every week, as a salesman. Like Willy Loman, sample cases in hand, he called on Macy's and Hutzler's, Abraham & Straus and Bloomingdale's, selling Arrow shirts, taking buyers out to dinner and drinks. As Willy says, the success of a salesman depends on being liked. My father was successful.

He was also fiercely independent once he retired. He and my

mother lived at home well into their eighties, and his job, in retirement, was taking care of her. As he eventually accepted the
need for care, the house filled up with nurse's aides and hospice
workers, visiting nurses and social workers. He managed to find humor in the situation, joking as he answered the phone, "Bouton
Nursing Home."

He didn't like the phone. If he answered when you called, you
were lucky to get three sentences: "Hey! How you? Your mother's
right here . . ." The sicker he got, the weaker his voice got and the less
I could hear him. His main concern about dying was what would
happen to my mother—his "bride." Corny but sweet. At eighty-six,
she had back problems, heart problems, memory problems. He took
care of her on his own long after his cancer diagnosis. During my
visits, he'd draw me aside, hoping my mother wouldn't hear his wor-
ries, but not a word escaped her, even when she was in another room.
If we talked about the possibility of her moving north with me, she'd
shout from the other room, "I want to stay right here."

Just before my father died, I called to say I was flying down the
next day. The nurse held the phone to his ear. "I love you, Dad," I
said, "I'll see you tomorrow." As I waited for the nurse to take back
the phone, I heard his voice, barely audible: "See you soon." At least
that's what I think he said.

• • •

I got married at twenty, unwisely, to my high school boyfriend.
We split up five tearful years later. I went from my unhappy marriage into a difficult and tumultuous romance with someone involved with someone else. It was the seventies, and to get back at
the man I wanted, I had casual retributive sex with other men.
I discovered opera, full-blown melodramatic Italian opera, listening to *La Bohème* and *La Traviata*, music that elevated my own
unhappy life into tragic romance.

I worked at *The New Yorker*. I had walked in one afternoon,
résumé in hand, and said I was looking for a job in magazine

design. At *The New Yorker*, that department was called Makeup, and it was all men. Would I like to apply for the typing pool instead? It paid $106 a week.

There were a dozen of us in the typing pool, known as Walden Pond after Harriet Walden, the fifty-ish supervisor who hired the young women (and later young men) who constituted the lowest of the editorial ranks at the magazine.

We typed. We typed handwritten manuscripts from writers who didn't know how to type. We typed revised manuscripts. We typed edited manuscripts. We typed and retyped. We filled in for absent secretaries and receptionists, which meant we met everyone who came and went. We were young, well educated, and available. Life at *The New Yorker* as I remember it in those years was one long flirtation.

As assistants and receptionists, we overheard and couldn't help seeing what went on around us. Senior editors and writers and cartoonists had affairs with each other and with us. Some of them drank too much. They married and remarried, sometimes each other. Maeve Brennan, an Irish redhead and alcoholic, and a venerable Talk of the Town writer (where she was known as the Long-Winded Lady), slept occasionally in the nineteenth-floor ladies' room on a couch tucked away in an anteroom. Her former husband, St. Clair McKelway, also an alcoholic, was said to have thrown a chair through an office door.

William Shawn, the august editor-in-chief, was famously eccentric. He was known as a devoted husband and father, yet he also had a decades-long relationship with the staff writer Lillian Ross, which she later wrote about in *Here but Not Here*. We'd see her in the office with her little poodle, Goldie, going in to visit Mr. Shawn. Sometimes she would come to the office with Erik, the tall, handsome son she adopted in Norway—who we fantasized was actually Mr. Shawn's son. (Given the almost uncanny family resemblance in Shawn's sons Wallace and Allen, who have the same sloped shoulders, round faces, and short legs as their father, this seems unlikely.)

The *New Yorker* offices had doors, which could be closed. The hotel down the street, then a dive, had a steamy reputation: "lunch at the Royalton" had a different meaning then. A charming and funny cartoonist (married) left flirtatious drawings on my desk. An editor twenty years my senior (also married) suggested we take a day off and go somewhere and have sex all day long, an idea that terrified me. (We didn't.) Meanwhile, I flirted with Dan Menaker, who was then a copy editor.

Every February, *The New Yorker* had a party to celebrate its anniversary, at a ballroom like the St. Regis Roof or the Plaza. Food and drink were plentiful, and there was always a band. Spouses were not invited. After one party in 1974, Dan and I shared a taxi back to the West Side. He held my hand. That was it. Not even a kiss. I left my husband six months later. Dan was in a long-term relationship with someone but we dated sporadically, intensely at times, neurotically always. I listened to tragic operas and wept. Finally, in 1977, as my thirtieth birthday approached, I moved in with him. Six months later I left for Turkey.

• • •

Even after the episode of my hearing loss, although I took time out for doctors' visits and an MRI, I kept writing compulsively about my trip to Turkey. A few months later, without so much as a by-your-leave, I handed Mr. Shawn an eighteen-thousand-word manuscript and asked if he would read it. He looked surprised, but accepted the pages I had in my hand. Two days later, he came back to me. "This is very good," he said, adding that he thought I needed to add a passage about such and such. "And, Miss Bouton," he said, "don't ever do this again." Next time, ask first.

The article appeared in the magazine as "A Reporter at Large" in 1978, my first *New Yorker* byline. I was thrilled. And the check seemed huge. I gave a portion of the proceeds to the New York Public Library—the first time in my life I had enough money to give some away.

Later I proposed other stories, some of which Mr. Shawn published and others which he bought and, to my frustration, held indefinitely. (He was so possessive about writers that this was a regular practice. When I left *The New Yorker*, there were some two hundred nonfiction pieces on the magazine's bank of stories to be published. The introduction to the *New Yorker* archives at the New York Public Library says that some stories were held for as long as twenty years before they were reedited and published, or killed. One such story of mine, on the bank for a mere three or four years, was later repurposed as a cover story for *The New York Times Magazine*.)

In the fall of 1979, a year and a half after my initial hearing loss, Mr. Shawn let me accept a National Science Foundation grant to travel to Antarctica. I wrote about it in a piece that ran in the magazine under the title "South of 60 Degrees South." I also sold some fiction to *The New Yorker*. One of my fellow Antarctic travelers was the NPR science journalist Ira Flatow. When we met afterward, he mentioned to my husband that he thought I was having trouble hearing. I knew that, of course, but I was embarrassed to realize that he did.

In February 1980, Dan and I got married. I think I heard my wedding vows: the chapel was an intimate space, and I was only half deaf then. We wanted to have children and set about trying. All too soon, it became clear we couldn't. Several years of fertility problems, three tries at IVF, surgeries, grief, anger—hearing issues were easily eclipsed.

In many ways, infertility is like hearing loss. The sufferer is reluctant to acknowledge it publicly. The terms used to describe it are harsh: "barren," "sterile." I kept my reproductive problems a secret, even through three catastrophically terminated pregnancies, each involving a week in the hospital. Only my closest friends knew. Much later, when I began to mourn my hearing loss, I at last allowed myself to mourn my lost fertility, and my lost babies as well.

At the time, though, I shoved grief aside. Dan and I started the adoption procedure, another distraction from hearing issues. Our son, William, was born in August 1983; our daughter, Elizabeth, in November 1986. We adopted each of them as infants—Elizabeth was just three days old; Will was twenty days old. They were the silver lining of my infertility, the blessing that would not have been without that grievous experience.

Did I hear their first words? Does anybody really hear when "ma-ma-ma" and "ba-ba-ba" turn into Mama and Dada? I remember two-year-old Will pointing his chubby finger and saying, "What's dat?" Then, later, "backhoe," "front loader," "construction site." As for Elizabeth, a feisty girl right from the start and tormented by her brother: "Don't bother me. Leave my lone."

As they got older, I heard less and less. I had trouble at teacher's conferences. One of the kids or my husband would fill me in. I missed most of what was said in school assemblies. I never heard a single graduation speech. There were times when my hearing loss was wrenching. I missed confidences, murmured fears, muttered anger. I never heard the backseat chatter and gossip between my children and their friends.

In 1988, when I was forty and my children were two and five, I went to work at *The New York Times Magazine* as an editor. I wore a headset for the phone, I worked with writers sitting on my right, and I always ensured that I was in the best position to hear at meetings. My colleagues at the magazine and in the various departments I worked in over the next two decades (science and the Sunday *New York Times Book Review*, bookended by two stints at the magazine) may well have known about my hearing loss, but we never spoke about it and I never acknowledged it.

• • •

Diane Ackerman, in *A Natural History of the Senses*, parses the origins of the word "absurdity," derived from the Latin word *absurdus*. *Absurdus* means out of tune or silly or senseless, and comes from *ab* ("away from") and *surdus* ("deafness"). She goes on to write, "The assumption in this etymological nest of spiders is that the world will still make sense to someone who is blind or armless or minus a nose. But if you lose your sense of hearing, a crucial thread dissolves and you lose track of life's logic." I think she's wrong on this: life's logic *can* make itself apparent, even to the deaf.

But I can't disagree with her next thought: "Sounds thicken the sensory stew of our lives, and we depend on them to help us interpret, communicate with, and express the world around us."

I hear voices, but I don't always hear words. Speech is visual. I read lips, I respond to gestures and body language. My mind supplies the words I don't get—or sometimes it doesn't. My son and his girlfriend were moving. "She'll have to give up Nona," Dan said. "Nona?" A grandmother? A dog? What? "She'll have to give up Nona," he repeated. He has trouble remembering the need to rephrase. What he might have said the second (and third and fourth) time was "She'll have to give up the place where she takes yoga." Context is everything.

So is close attention to the speaker. Jess Dancer, an emeritus professor of audiology at the University of Arkansas, recently noted that "it's not unusual for speech intelligibility to increase from 20 percent when listening in noise without vision, to 80 percent or more when the speaker is seen as well as heard." Writing in an on-line professional hearing journal, he went on: "This four-fold performance improvement is based upon the principle of 'bisensory integration,' in which combining two senses produce[s] more information together than would be predicted from merely adding the performance of the two senses separately."

"Bisensory integration" is also known as the McGurk (or McGurk-Macdonald) effect, after the two scientists who first happened on the discovery in 1976 that speech perception is multimodal. I'm a fair lip-reader, but I am a very attentive listener. Like many hearing-impaired people, I intuitively practice the McGurk effect—"hearing lips and seeing voices," as they put it. This bimodal effect can also be achieved by reading captions or lyrics while listening.

Dancer feels that paying attention to the speaker is far more important than structured lipreading. Speechreading (the correct term these days) was the core curricular component at schools for the deaf until well into the twentieth century, when American Sign Language was finally recognized as a mode of communication. At the Center for Hearing and Communication in Manhattan (formerly the League for the Hard of Hearing), speechreading is an integral part of hearing rehabilitation.

I'd like to be a more fluent speech-reader, but the courses are time-consuming and the results varied. I was tempted after reading about the professional lip-reader Tina Lannin, deaf from birth, who managed to pick up much of the (predictable) conversation between Kate Middleton and Prince William at the royal wedding. "You look beautiful," William said to Kate at the altar, later asking her several times if she was okay. The Queen, however, sounded peevish when she was "overheard" by Lannin saying: "I wanted them to take the smaller carriage."

Even face-to-face, and with training, lipreading can be difficult. Researchers estimate that only 40 percent of the sounds of speech are visible on the lips. The letters *b*, *m*, and *p* look exactly the same. Then there are those troublesome mustaches and beards, or people who speak with their hands in front of their mouths, ashamed of their teeth perhaps, or while chewing, or looking down at their BlackBerry or rummaging in their purse. Oliver Sacks quotes a deaf woman in *The Mind's Eye* who reads lips. When he turns his head away from her while talking, she says, "I can't hear you."

I have the great advantage of having heard for most of my life, which means I know what language sounds like and I can put the sounds I hear together with the sounds I expect to hear. It's the unexpected that trips me up. Out walking with my dog, people ask, "How old is he?" "What kind of dog is he?" "What's his name?" The questions are all the same length, and caught in the rustle of wind and the hum from the West Side Highway, they all sound the same to me. How old is he? Tibetan Terrier. What kind of dog is he? A year and a half. What's his name? I usually get that one right. But when I reciprocate, "What's your dog's name?" Marley comes out as Paulie, then Barley; Fargo as Margo; Morris as Norris, Moreth, Norman, Mormon, etc.

Dan likes to talk in non sequiturs—his mind tends to race and he enjoys wordplay and leapfrogging through thoughts in conversation. I'm totally lost. In a noisy place—a dinner party, the street, a restaurant, the lobby of a theater, a waiting room with a television on, my book club, a room with a noisy air conditioner—I can't pick up even the expected.

I've often wondered if I hear in my dreams. I sense that I hear voices, tone and pitch and intonation, as precisely as I once did. In dreams, it turns out, I am on level ground with those who hear. "When we hear voices, spoken language, in dreams," Freud writes in *The Interpretation of Dreams*, "we are all abnormal in the sense that there is no actual source of sound around; all the voices are silently generated by our minds, not by some external entity."

Sometimes I take my hearing aid and implant off and just relax into silence. Wearing them is tiring. Listening is exhausting. From the time I turn out the light till daybreak, I am essentially blind and deaf. My husband acts as my eyes and ears when he's around. My dog fills in when he's not. He barks when someone knocks on the door or, at our house in the country, when someone comes up the driveway. But like many people with hearing loss, I feel vulnerable at night. I think I would hear the smoke alarm right over the bed. I think the dog would bark or jump on me if someone tried to break in. I hope. There are devices designed for people with hearing loss—alarm systems that work with vibration or strobe lights—but for the moment I'm taking the low-tech dog route. (As it turned out, this too was a form of denial. See the last paragraph in the notes for this chapter on page 249.)

What do we hear when there's nothing at all to hear? George Prochnik, the author of *In Pursuit of Silence*, went in search of the quietest place in the world and eventually found himself in the basement sanctuary of the Trappist New Melleray Abbey, in Iowa. The monk who showed him the way warned him, Prochnik writes, "that the silence of the room was so intense that it was likely to 'take me outside of my comfort zone.'" Some people from big cities, the monk added, find themselves "physically unable to remain in the chapel for even five minutes."

As it turned out, it wasn't as quiet as it might have been. There was another monk in the room, "a large man sitting with his legs wide apart and his hands on his thighs, breathing quite loudly." But that doesn't seem to have disturbed Prochnik's sense of the deep silence. The monks, he observed, listen to silence for self-knowledge. Far from being out of his comfort zone, he was disappointed when it was time to leave.

Prochnik doesn't describe what silence sounds like, but I can. It's noisy. The brain creates noise to fill the silence, and we hear this as tinnitus. Perhaps only someone with profound deafness can achieve this level of silence, so paradoxically loud. As Brad May, a professor of otolaryngology and head and neck surgery at Johns Hopkins University, explained to me, once the auditory machinery that would ordinarily be transmitting sound to the brain stops working, the synaptic balance in those neurons goes haywire, because nothing is regulating it, "nothing is pulling it down into its proper level of activity." And so the brain starts generating its own activity in that pathway, and the result can be ringing, or buzzing, or humming—all of which fall under the catchall term "tinnitus." Sylvia, in Nina Raine's *Tribes*, says of going deaf, "No one told me it was going to be this *noisy* . . . It's this buzz. This roar and outside . . . it's all—black."

I have it easy, and in fact kind of like my tinnitus: it changes pitch from time to time, an ethereal deep outer space keening.

· · ·

Anatomically, the inner ear is one of the most inaccessible areas of the body. In addition, the structure of the inner ear is complex, delicate, and well protected by its bony casing. The result is that we know very little about what goes on there. As the Stanford University researcher Stefan Heller wrote in 2010, "We continue to lack nondestructive means of diagnosing or manipulating specific pathology for even the most common disorders."

I spent years requesting tests and searching out far-fetched explanations. I repeatedly asked my ENT doctor, Ronald Hoffman, if there wasn't another test or procedure we could try. Not impatiently, but with a certain weariness, he said, "We could do an autopsy." An autopsy may well explain what went wrong in my inner ear, and why. But for now I am left with "idiopathic," a word that sounds uncomfortably like "idiot," which is how you often feel when you have hearing loss.

VOICES: BEN LUXON

The British opera singer Ben Luxon denied his hearing loss until he couldn't anymore. That moment happened to be during a recital. The program was a Schubert cycle. "I sang the first song," he told me. "I could see from people's faces . . . hmmm . . . something's not good here, and then the second song, I couldn't even start. This was the pattern for the next five or six songs, until at last I just had to stop and say to people, 'I can't submit you or myself to this any longer, something is seriously wrong with my hearing,' and so that was that. That was on a Friday evening . . ." By Sunday he was totally deaf in one ear and sound was seriously distorted in the other.

I visited Luxon in his comfortable kitchen in rural Massachusetts, birds on the feeder just outside the window. Luxon had continued to sing for some time, he said that day, even after he began to notice that things seemed out of whack. He was cast as Papageno in *The Magic Flute* for the English National Opera. During rehearsals the conductor mentioned that his voice was "a little sharp" in places, just above the correct pitch, but ENO wanted him to do the role anyway. "I couldn't hear the orchestra—the orchestra sounded like people banging on big iron pipes in the bottom of a pit, it was just so distorted," he said. "And the soprano, when I was singing the duet with her, that beautiful duet in Act 1, once she got above an F or G, her voice split like a cat yowling. It went in two directions, and I thought, 'My God, this is really wild, bizarre.'"

A few months later, he was scheduled to sing the Schubert recital. Warming up before the concert, he said to the pianist, "I have no idea . . . I can't hear where the pitch is." He didn't know where to sing. He stood beside the keyboard; he tried standing at the end of the piano; he moved around, looking for the maximum connection with the sounds from the piano. They went ahead with the concert anyway: "I thought for the concert, with a little adrenaline I'd probably be okay."

He spent the following year being treated with steroids and a treatment involving chemotherapy. He got a hearing aid, and with 55 percent of the hearing left in his other ear, went back to his professional career on a reduced schedule. Eventually, after another two years, the stress and isolation of not being able to hear what was going on around him in a performance proved too daunting. He stopped singing.

These days, he's turned to recitations and acting. To anticipate his cues, he roughly memorizes the whole play, so he can "feel" the length of speeches. We talked that afternoon for several hours, and quite often, to illustrate a point, he would break into song—a Rex Harrison half-singing/half-talking voice rather than his full-throttle operatic voice. With the aid of a cochlear implant and a hearing aid, in addition to his recitations and acting, he also teaches.

Luxon said he can hear the quality of a voice—he can tell whether a singer is using the voice properly, breathing properly, and so on—but not the pitch. "I had a lesson this morning with a very good singer, very nice. And so I'm perfectly fine, I play the piano as well. Hearing harmonics on the piano is difficult and I can play wrong notes all over the place, but I'm usually blissfully unaware."

Luxon and his wife, Susie Crofut, have created a magical garden around their big house, which is a welcoming sprawl of rooms. On the day I visited, the house was full of children and grandchildren from their combined families. Susie's late husband, the singer and composer Bill Crofut, whose music encompassed jazz and folk, had as part of his eclectic career collaborated with Ben, among other classical musicians. It is a musical family, and Ben participates in family music-making, but not using his operatic voice.

"I hear the birds," he said. "I was sitting out on the deck the other day, it was so beautiful, and there was this damn bird that was going [he imitates the bird whistle], so I can hear the pitch and imitate it pretty accurately, but I couldn't locate the bird. I didn't know where to look."

He laughed as he told me this, his Cornish accent and cheerful, resilient personality making everything seem really, actually, not so bad. "Location is gone, for anything . . . If I hear Susie calling . . . sometimes I get flashes of mini-fury, 'For God's sake! Where are you? Are you bloody well upstairs or downstairs!'" He laughs again. "That's a funny one."

He told me he had worked with a man in Boston named Geoff Plant, who had helped him recover his speech perception. Plant often works with musicians. "We did an experiment where I tried to sing properly with fairly full voice, and I sang all over the place. But then, if I sang lightly and fairly quickly, I sang in tune. I was convinced I was singing in tune both times." He urged me to visit Plant, and to watch him work.

Ben Luxon has suffered a major setback; his singing career is over, the turn his professional life has taken is permanent. But of all the people I met while researching this book, he is the only one— myself included, I think—who has truly come to that elusive state of acceptance.

TWO

Why?

There's a joke about hearing loss: A man tells his doctor he thinks his wife is losing her hearing. "Try this test to find out for sure," the doctor says. "When your wife is in the kitchen doing dishes, stand fifteen feet behind her and ask her a question. If she doesn't respond, keep moving closer and repeat the question until she hears you." The man goes home and stands fifteen feet behind his wife and says, "What's for dinner, honey?" He gets no response, so he moves to ten feet behind her and asks again. Still no response, so he moves to five feet. Again, no answer. Finally he stands directly behind her and says, "Honey, what's for supper?" She replies, "For the fourth time, I SAID CHICKEN!!"

There are two types of hearing loss: conductive and sensorineural. Sensorineural damage accounts for 90 percent of all hearing loss, and is usually the result of aging or noise exposure. It is most often caused by damage to the tiny hair cells in the inner ear. Sometimes the damage is to the auditory nerve, which carries sound to the brain. Sensorineural loss (usually referred to as SNHL, or SSNHL when it comes on suddenly) is rarely reversible.

In children, the most common kind of acquired hearing loss is conductive. It can be caused by something as simple as wax buildup in the ear or as complicated as a structural anomaly. Wax can usually be easily removed by a doctor. Trying to get it out yourself with a Q-tip only serves to impact it. The same is true for "foreign bodies," as the medical literature puts it, in the external ear canal (marbles, toys, anything that a child, or even an adult, might stick into the ear), which can also usually be removed in an office procedure. An infection in the outer ear canal, which can cause temporary conductive hearing loss, is painful and visible.

Middle ear conductive loss can be caused by chronic otitis media, with the classic symptoms of an earache, a common problem in children. Children with chronic ear infections are often treated with ear tubes, surgically inserted into the eardrum, to drain fluid buildup. They need to be replaced as the child grows.

Conductive hearing loss can also be the result of a perforated eardrum, caused by diving, a sudden change in air pressure, or exposure to a sudden loud noise. All are painful. Some cure themselves. Some don't. Finally, conductive hearing loss can be caused by otosclerosis, structural damage like a bony growth or tumors in the middle ear. Sometimes it can be treated surgically. Sometimes hearing aids help.

• • •

Although hearing loss is an age-related condition, you don't have to be old to have hearing loss, as the 2010 study in *The Journal of the American Medical Association* (which found hearing loss in 19.5 percent of the twelve-to-nineteen-year-olds studied) demonstrates. Eighteen percent of American adults forty-five to sixty-four years old, 30 percent of adults sixty-five to seventy-four years old, and 47 percent of adults seventy-five years old or older have a hearing impairment. If you live into your eighties, that number jumps to 90 percent, according to a February 2011 study. (My mother, in her late eighties with acute hearing, is part of a very small minority.) Cardiovascular disease is strongly correlated with low-frequency hearing loss. The explanation is that the thickening of the arteries that causes heart disease may also contribute to hearing loss.

Hearing impairment is usually described in terms of the degree of impairment, ranging from mild to moderate to severe to profound. In order to understand how hearing loss is quantified, you have to understand how hearing loss is measured. To understand how hearing is measured, you have to understand what a decibel is. One decibel (abbreviated dB) is the just noticeable difference (louder or softer) between sound pressure levels. A 1-decibel decrease produces a sound that is just noticeably softer than the previous sound.

The softest sound a person can hear is called their hearing threshold. For people with mild hearing loss, the hearing threshold—that is, the lowest decibel level at which they can hear sounds—ranges between 26 and 40 decibels.

If they can't hear until the dB level is raised to between 41 and 55 dB, their loss is classified as moderate. A moderately *severe* loss is between 56 and 70 dBs. A severe loss is between 71 and 90 dBs. (The hearing in my right ear, the good one, measures between 70 in the low frequencies down to the 90s in the high frequencies. This explains why I can hear thunder but not a siren.) If you can't hear at 91 dBs, you are considered profoundly deaf. Hearing loss in any one individual affects some frequencies more than others. In most people with SNHL, the higher frequencies go first. Speech falls in the mid-to-high-frequency range, the so-called banana on an audiogram, which encompasses the speech frequencies. This is why even people with mild hearing loss have problems with speech perception.

This threshold naturally begins to rise (in other words, your hearing begins to deteriorate) in your thirties. Sharon Kujawa and Charles Liberman, in the Department of Otology and Laryngology at Harvard Medical School, believe this deterioration is a combination of the effect of aging and exposure to noise.

• • •

Ototoxins—diseases, drugs, or conditions that destroy hearing—include drugs like Cisplatin and Vicodin, autoimmune diseases like lupus and Lyme disease, viruses, acoustic neuroma, Ménière's disease, and—by far the most common—exposure to either long-term moderately loud noise or sudden very loud noise. How is it that these varied elements can do such similar damage to the inner ear hair cells or to the nerves that transmit the sound to the brain? What's the common factor? What actually happens in the inner ear when it is exposed to ototoxins or loud noise?

The inner ear is home to the cochlea, a bony spiral cavity about the size of a pea, which turns on itself two and a half times and looks like a snail shell ("cochlea" comes from the Latin term for "snail"). Sound waves, or vibrations, enter the cochlea (having been given a boost by the middle ear's three interconnected bones, including the stapes, the smallest bone in the body). As this happens, fluid in the cochlea sets in motion the thousands of hair cells located in the organ of Corti, deep in the inner ear.

The hair cells in the organ of Corti are organized into four rows. The three outer rows of cells pick up the movement and change it into a mechanical impulse, which amplifies the signal—now traveling through the cochlear bath and thus dulled, as sound would be if you were underwater. The inner hair cells, in a single row, each respond to a particular frequency. They are activated to release a neurotransmitter to the auditory nerve fibers, which also number in the thousands and also each respond to a different frequency. The neurons transmit the sound via the auditory nerve to the brain, ultimately reaching the auditory cortex, which translates the sound into something that we recognize as speech or birdsong or a car passing on the road. The translation that occurs in the auditory cortex allows us to distinguish between similar speech sounds like "ah" and "eh," "b" and "p," "ch" and "sh." How the cortex does this is beyond the scope of this book. Suffice it to say that you hear with your brain. The auditory system merely transmits the signals. But if the signals can't get to the brain, then the brain can't do its job.

In a lot of deafness, the first things you lose are the outer hair cells. The inner hair cells may be undamaged, but because you've lost the mechanical response of the outer cells, the cochlea is not as sensitive, not as fine-tuned in its response. The result is that some neurons respond to more frequencies than they should, sending a muddled signal to the brain. The primary damage is to speech recognition. "Bet" sounds like "pet," "church" sounds like "shirts." Brad May, of Johns Hopkins, calls this "brain deafness." When I first got my cochlear implant, I practiced hearing, often with a friend who was recovering from cancer. She would read and I would try to understand what she was saying. I made many amusing mistakes. "Tiger Woods was tucked away, eating paper," I heard in a reading from *People* magazine. (He wasn't eating paper, he was reading *Playboy*.)

Outer cell damage can come from loud noise, certain viral infections, migraine, ototoxic drugs, and aging. These types of hearing loss are often referred to as nerve damage but they are not, technically, since they don't affect the acoustic nerve, only the hair cells that communicate with it. True nerve damage can be caused by an acoustic neuroma or viral infections like herpes zoster, or shingles, which can also kill hair cells. Sometimes aging results in nerve damage as well as hair cell damage.

The results of hair cell damage, according to Brad May, are insidious: "I can hear you speak but I cannot understand what you're saying. So the problem is not about a loss of hearing sensitivity, for most impaired listeners. It is a loss of frequency tuning that is the big problem." Although high frequencies usually are the first to go, most people don't realize they have a hearing problem until lower speech frequencies are affected. May's multidisciplinary approach to hearing loss reflects his academic background: a B.A. in zoology from Indiana University, a Ph.D. in biopsychology from the University of Michigan, a postdoctoral degree in biomedical engineering from Hopkins.

A person with mild to moderate hearing loss can still hear in a quiet room or other favorable environment. But when too many frequencies are destroyed, he or she may not understand speech, even under the best of conditions.

The muddled transmissions also make it difficult for the auditory system to filter unwanted noise: the din and clatter of a restaurant, the engine of a bus, the hum of a fan or air conditioner. Intrusive noise may be simply two or three people talking at once, creating a background sound of indistinguishable voices, or it may be a large, resonant room echoing sound off the walls. Or maybe all it takes is one other person near you talking loudly, drowning out the person you're with. (When my father was sick, I couldn't hear him over the oxygen machine.) All of these get in the way of the one thing you want to hear: the speaker's voice. What hearing aids do is amplify the sound—the sound per se becomes easier to hear. But since hearing aids aren't as good as the human ear at screening out unwanted noise, using them can be frustrating, especially in noisy environments.

• • •

Assuming my hair cells are damaged, they probably look flattened, like a field of wheat after a hailstorm, as Sharon Kujawa put it in a talk at the 2011 meeting of the Hearing Loss Association of America (HLAA). Each cell in those four rows of cells (the single inner row, which communicates with the brain, and three outer rows) is topped by a tiny standing hair, or stereocilium. The hair cells, she said, are "connected to each other with fine little filaments, so that when sound comes in and they bend, it allows currents to flow through." This movement triggers the release of the neurotransmitter substances. After intense noise exposure, the hair cells lie flat. If the noise is not too loud, they eventually right themselves: The threshold shift is temporary.

But Kujawa and Liberman have found that even though the threshold reverts to normal, permanent damage may have occurred. Studies on mice show an alarming relationship between persistent exposure to even moderately loud noise and, decades later, an acceleration in presbycusis, the official term for age-related hearing loss. Kujawa and Liberman found that the damage occurs not in the hair cells themselves, which may recover, but in the spiral ganglion cells (SGCs—the cells in the cochlear neurons). The hair cells communicate with SGCs in the process of passing information to the brain.

Although hearing is restored, the damage is done almost instantaneously. As Kujawa and Liberman wrote in a 2009 paper, "The long-term fate of SGCs is sealed within the first twenty-four hours postexposure." The synapses between the hair cells and the nerves may be interrupted, even if the hair cells themselves are undamaged. The Harvard researchers believe that this synapse damage can lead to a number of perceptual problems, like difficulty hearing speech in noise, tinnitus, or hyperacusis (intolerance of noise).

Even though we think of this kind of hearing loss as related to aging, the truth is that ears are most vulnerable to noise damage when they're young. Kujawa and Liberman showed that in mice, the transition to tough ears happens around eight weeks. (The human equivalent would be around twenty years.) They note that mice reach sexual maturity around five weeks (females first, then males) and speculate that endocrine changes may affect cochlear function and influence noise vulnerability.

If these mouse findings are also true in humans, it means that teenagers—with their ubiquitous iPods and MP3 players, not to mention noise exposure from video games, loud stadiums, and rock concerts—are experiencing these loud noises at an especially vulnerable age.

• • •

Another vulnerable population, newborn infants, might suffer damage from continuous noise in a neonatal ICU or from a white noise machine parents sometimes use to help fussy infants sleep. Using mice again, Brad May and Amanda Lauer at Hopkins studied what happens in immature animals when the medial olivo-cochlear system (MOC) is weak or absent—something that is often missed in neonatal screening. They hypothesize that the function of the MOC system is to preserve normal development in the immature auditory system when it is challenged by continuous background noise.

To test this, they used mice in which they had switched off the MOC gene. "Noise-reared knock-out mice showed a decreased ability to process rapid acoustic events," they wrote in a 2011 paper. "Additional anatomical and physiological assessments linked these perceptual deficits to synaptic defects in the auditory brainstem." The mouse brain stem shares important features with that in humans. The Lauer and May paper raises critical questions about noise exposure for infants.

Most humans have intact MOC systems and are resistant to continuous noise. But some are born without this system fully intact. Although all newborns are screened for hearing loss, a weak MOC system would not show up in routine neonatal testing. If these infants happened to be exposed to noise in the neonatal intensive care unit (this group, of course, would have other, more visible and urgent problems) or to a white noise machine, they would be at risk for a condition known as auditory neuropathy.

White noise, May explained, "has all of the frequencies in it, so it's causing everything to fire all the time; there is no exclusive kind of response. When that happens, you don't have a strengthening of some synapses and a weakening of others, so the auditory system is not able to process information. It is able to hear, to detect sound, but it can't discriminate one sound from another."

The damage becomes evident only when a child begins to have problems in school or in learning to speak. An audiogram shows that they have normal hearing, but, May said, "if they do a more sophisticated kind of test they would see that this child doesn't process language. The reason the child doesn't process language is because he or she doesn't code the timing of sound very well." This condition, auditory neuropathy, is not well understood. Lauer and May's experiment provided the first animal model of how it might occur.

• • •

People are affected to different degrees by noise exposure. Some seem simply to have genetically tough ears, others weak ones. As Kujawa and Liberman have hypothesized, noise exposure in some cases can lead to accelerated or early-onset presbycusis. In fact, as Liberman told me in an interview at Harvard (Sharon Kujawa was out of town), he wonders if all age-related hearing loss isn't actually accumulated noise-related loss.

There have been several studies of populations in areas where there is very little noise: Easter Island is one, parts of the Sudan another. Researchers in the Sudan, Liberman told me, find that even people over a hundred years old often have perfect hearing. A study of adult Easter Islanders with perfect hearing found that they began to suffer hearing loss within a few years of emigrating to the far noisier industrialized environment of Chile. Such studies are "proof that it is possible for the ear to live and function for a hundred years and not fall apart," Liberman said. One possible conclusion is that the absence of noise results in an absence of noise-related hearing loss.

But it's not that simple. This phenomenon "doesn't mean that if you and I move to Sudan, we'll have the same experience. There are genetic differences, obviously," Liberman says. "It could be that these Sudan tribesmen have a gene that protects their inner ears. We know that there is a huge genetic component to resistance and vulnerability of the ear, and it's true in acoustic trauma too."

Frank Lin, the epidemiologist at Johns Hopkins, has documented an interesting genetic pattern to hearing resistance. One risk factor for hearing loss is the color of your skin. The lighter your skin, the higher your risk. "Light-skinned whites are at highest risk. Being black is determined by skin color, by the melanin in the skin," he explained. "Melanin also exists in the inner ear. There is likely concordance in the amount of melanin in the skin and the inner ear— the darker your skin, the more pigment in the inner ear. Melanin may serve as a kind of free radical scavenger and help protect the inner ear from damage over time."

This is not only a curious fact but also a clue to a potential therapy, which could lead to a pharmacological target. "Synthetic analogs of melanocyte-stimulating hormone already exist," Lin said. "Could this possibly be used to help delay or reduce hearing loss in older adults? There have been a couple of animal studies that suggest this might be possible. When animals were pre-treated with melanocyte-stimulating hormone and then given a drug that is toxic to the inner ear, the animals treated with drug versus placebo were actually somewhat protected against hearing loss and inner ear damage."

Unfortunately, though, these pieces of evidence for a protective association between pigmentation and hearing loss often go unnoticed by most hearing scientists, Lin said. "As a whole, studying age-related hearing loss and how to prevent it is not a priority, because it's still perceived as being an inconsequential part of aging."

• • •

The fact that not everyone exposed to ototoxins ends up with hearing loss also suggests a protective genetic component. Neil G. Bauman's *Ototoxic Drugs Exposed: The Shocking Truth About Prescription Drugs, Medications, Chemicals and Herbals That Can (and Do) Damage Our Ears* (now in its third edition) includes 798 pages of information about every drug that may (or may not) cause hearing loss. They include painkillers like Vicodin and Oxy-Contin as well as aspirin and ibuprofen in large doses, which can result in temporary or permanent loss. The chemotherapy drug Cisplatin is known to be a powerful ototoxin, as are some classes of antibiotics, loop diuretics, and quinine. Dr. Neil, as he likes to be called, is a perennially popular speaker at hearing loss conventions and the author of many books, including, *Help! I'm Losing My Hearing—What Do I Do Now?*

Rarely, sensorineural hearing loss can be a symptom of any one of dozens of syndromes, usually characterized by other obvious abnormalities. These include Usher and Pendred syndromes, both of which have other visible and debilitating physiological manifestations.

Seventy percent of genetic hearing loss is hereditary. This may not always be apparent, with the genetic defect either skipping generations or carried by someone who died too young to reach the age when hearing loss might begin to be recognized. Hearing loss can occur at any time. For males, the peak age of onset is between the ages of twenty and fifty-nine, accounting for 64 percent of all men with hearing loss. For females, onset is evenly distributed over the decades.

Sudden sensorineural hearing loss can be the result of exposure to an explosion or other literally deafening noise. But the cause may be invisible—a genetic weakness, triggered by exposure to an ototoxin. Sudden sensorineural hearing loss may be immediately severe or even profound, or it may be inexorably progressive. Mine is the latter. By definition, sudden sensorineural hearing loss is hearing loss greater than 30 dB over three contiguous pure-tone frequencies, occurring within a three-day period. Usually it affects just one ear, and sometimes it can be reversed.

Sudden and progressive is not an unusual combination. My hearing loss fluctuates, but in the end it always fluctuates downward. Although certainly there are scores of possible causes of sudden deafness, only 10 to 15 percent of patients ever discover what went wrong. The cause is unknown—that distressing word "idiopathic."

• • •

The pattern of my loss, as seen on an audiogram, rules out noise damage, despite The Who at Madison Square Garden. An audiogram done in my thirties shows normal hearing in my right ear: a steady horizontal line left to right, from the low frequencies to the high. The pattern for my left ear, on the other hand, is jagged, beginning with moderate loss in the low frequencies, peaking briefly in the mid-level frequencies at mild loss, and then plunging in the high frequencies (the 4000-to-6000-hertz range) to severe to profound. The audiogram pattern looks a little like the Matterhorn.

Noise-induced loss tends to be steady across all frequencies. The Matterhorn pattern showed that my loss was not caused by noise. The mid-to-high-frequency loss meant that I had very compromised ability to hear conversation in my left ear. But my right ear compensated. The primary speech areas of the brain, at least in terms of grammar and vocabulary, are in the left brain, and this may have helped me. I've often wondered: If the more severe loss had been in my right ear, would my left ear have had a harder time catching up? The left and right hemispheres are permeable, but the right is less focused on vocabulary and more on intonation and context, as well as on analytical skills.

I've had three MRIs over three decades, which have repeatedly ruled out an acoustic neuroma. A CT scan ruled out vestibular disease. I might have Ménière's, which is itself an idiopathic condition, a diagnosis that is often made when all other causes have been ruled out. There is currently no test for Ménière's except to examine the inner ear on autopsy, as my ENT doctor so helpfully suggested. I wasn't ready for an autopsy yet. The symptoms of Ménière's include hearing loss (usually but not always on one side), periodic episodes of vertigo (which I developed only in my sixties), tinnitus, and a sensation of fullness or pressure in the ears.

The vertigo of Ménière's is caused by fluid buildup in the inner ear. When this fluid builds up, it can rupture the membrane separating the two chambers of the ear, allowing the potassium-rich endolymph to combine with the fluid next door, the potassium-poor perilymph. The chemical mixture creates havoc. It coats the vestibular nerves, making them dysfunctional.

In a search for the explanation for my hearing loss, I've been tested for every known autoimmune disorder. ("Known" is the key word in that sentence. There are more than eighty known auto-immune disorders, and many are difficult to diagnose.) I could have a form of migraine (without a headache), but my vertigo is of recent onset and is only somewhat exacerbated by bright lights or loud noises, and, like Ménière's, migraine usually results in hearing loss in only one ear. I've had dozens of viral tests over the years. I don't take Vicodin or any medication in large doses. I've never been treated with Cisplatin or any other ototoxic medication. I've had measles, mumps, scarlet fever, and repeated infections in childhood that resulted in having my tonsils out at five, but none of these cause hearing loss that manifests itself twenty-five years later.

I cast about for answers, trying one search term after another on the Internet, asking every doctor I meet for new ideas. At one point I enlisted the help of Lisa Sanders, who writes *The Times Magazine*'s Diagnosis column and is a dogged researcher when presented with an intractable problem. She came up with the same frustrating nothing. (Dr. Sanders's column was the inspiration for *House*, and she was medical adviser to the show. I'm sure Dr. House could figure out my hearing loss.)

John Oghalai, part of the Stanford School of Medicine's Initiative to Cure Hearing Loss, points out that an accurate diagnosis eludes most sensorineural hearing loss. I visited him in the spring of 2012 at Stanford, the prosperous campus bursting with spring flowers abutting vast construction projects. Stanford has an ambitious and well-funded otolaryngology department, where some of the country's most important research on finding a biological cure for hearing loss is going on.

Oghalai was telling me about a device his lab is developing to look inside the human cochlea to find out exactly what's causing an individual's hearing loss. I asked whether the device would be able to see my damaged hair cells. "Who told you your hair cells were damaged?" he asked. I was taken aback. "Well, I have sensorineural hearing loss . . ."

"Has anybody seen your hair cells?" he asked, a rhetorical question since we both knew that the only way to see your hair cells is in an autopsy. "They may still be there," he said. "There are several other things that can go wrong in a cochlea besides hair cells. They may end up *causing* hair cell loss but it could be the nerve, it could be in some of the cells that produce endolymph, or some of the fluids in the cochlea. It could be some of the cells that support the hair cells."

Oghalai is in the process of developing a technique based on optical coherence tomography. He described it as being like ultrasound, but using laser light instead of ultrasonic waves, which allows much higher resolution. It's used already by ophthalmologists to look into the retina. The technique is noninvasive and the patient shouldn't feel anything.

He has built a prototype in a soundproof room, which he took me to see. The prototype, built principally by Simon Gao, a graduate student in engineering, was so big there was room only for a cramped desk in addition. Attached to the machine was a mouse (looking none too comfortable). Gao was peering at a computer screen, which showed the inner ear of the mouse. The structure dwarfed the mouse at about the same proportion that Macy's Herald Square (which bills itself as "The World's Largest Store") would dwarf me if I were standing on Thirty-fourth Street.

Within a year, Oghalai said, they hope to condense the hardware into a suitcase-size package that can be used by an otolaryngologist. That means that within a year, hearing loss like mine could be accurately described as inner or outer hair cell loss, neuron damage, supporting cell damage, and so on. The technique has already proved successful in mice and the concept has FDA approval. It won't diagnose all hearing damage, but it will help distinguish one inner ear problem from another. Once we understand what has gone wrong, we can begin to develop a diagnosis. Once we have a diagnosis, we can begin to work on a cure.

What will they call it? "I have no idea," Oghalai said. "Cochlear endoscopy? Or cochleoscope?"

I'd be first in line to volunteer for the cochleoscope. The longer I've had hearing loss and the more serious it has become, the more obsessed I am with finding the cause. Like many with undiagnosed hearing loss, I focus on finding an explanation as displacement for accepting the brutal reality that there is no cure.

. . .

Since no one else has an explanation, I've come up with one myself—far-fetched, one that I can neither prove nor disprove, but one that came to seem more plausible as I talked to various researchers around the country: I picked up something lethal to my hearing on that 1977 trip to Turkey, a parasite or a virus, which triggered a genetic flaw that led to my initial hearing loss.

That trip was exciting but physically grueling—three months in Turkey, working on a dig and traveling on the cheap. I was healthy when I went, unhealthy when I returned, and I lost my hearing four or five months later.

It was an adventure, an antidote to turning thirty. I'd worked for almost ten years at *The New Yorker* and thought that if I didn't get out and try my hand at reporting then, I'd be in an office for the rest of my life.

I flew to Athens on July 31, 1977, and turned thirty somewhere over the Atlantic. I had a round-trip ticket and $600 in traveler's checks, plus a vague arrangement with an archaeologist to help out at her excavation site on the southwest coast of Turkey and maybe to write about it.

The archaeologist was Iris Love—an apt name for someone who devoted decades to searching for a famed and long-lost statue of Aphrodite. This would be her tenth season excavating at the ancient city of Knidos and she invited me to be part of her team of volunteers.

The group would arrive at the site in the first week of August, she told me, gathering first in Bodrum, a seacoast town a few hours north, in late July. I could meet them in Bodrum or go straight to Knidos in early August. I planned to travel straight to Knidos, arriving on August 3, when the group should already have set up camp. The route would take me from Athens to Rhodes, and from there by a second ferry to a seaport on the southern coast of Turkey. Iris told me the overland portion of the trip once I arrived in Turkey would take six or seven hours, and gave me directions.

I had never traveled alone before, and Athens in August is daunting. Jet-lagged from the flight, I was overwhelmed by the heat and the traffic, the air pollution, the unreadable signs, the diesel-fueled buses and trucks. On later trips I would come to love Athens, walking everywhere, especially in the early morning when housewives and storekeepers scrub their sidewalks and the day feels fresh and new. But not that time.

On the overnight ferry to Rhodes I slept on the open deck in my borrowed blue cotton sleeping bag (not waterproof) and woke up soaked through with dew. From Rhodes I negotiated a ride to Marmaris, a resort on the Mediterranean. The official ferries were canceled because of a dispute between Greece and Turkey. A few other tourists and I traveled in a small open boat under the midday sun.

Marmaris was then a fishing village, and in early August it was also host to hordes of vacationers. The narrow beach was packed with Turkish families and a few European sunbathers, and was littered with corncobs (roasted corn on the cob being the local equivalent of the Coney Island hot dog). The next leg of my trip was by "taxi," to the inland town of Datca. The trip today, about fifty miles to Datca, takes just a couple of hours. Then it was four or five, over a narrow road that overhung the cliffs.

The only taxi had left for the day, so I found a small windowless room, possibly the only room in town still available. Later that day, walking on the beach, I fell into conversation with a German backpacker, who suggested we eat together at a seafront restaurant. Oblivious to the noxious potential, I had fish and a salad. A sleepless night, on the roof of the airless hotel with all the other guests, was punctuated by frequent trips to the shared hall toilet one flight down.

Early the next morning, I shouldered my backpack and found the taxi, a minivan with open sides, boxes and crates and chickens piled on top. "Hello," "Excuse me," "Thank you," straight from my little yellow Turkish phrasebook, as I climbed over plump old Turkish women and wizened old Turkish men until I found a space on a wooden bench.

At one point we stopped at a spring, where we drank from a communal tin cup hanging from a chain. From Datca I took an actual taxi, a tiny Fiat, to Knidos. Today the trip takes about forty-five minutes along a spectacular, and nerve-racking, coast route. In 1977, it was another two hours or so. A long, hot, and very dusty travel day.

We got to Knidos, the site of the excavation, in the late afternoon. Knidos is on a point of land overlooking the Aegean, at the tip of what is known as the Datca Peninsula. The island of Kos is visible offshore. An army garrison fronted the water, guns trained toward Greece. As we drove in, I saw caves in the hillside, temporary shelter for some of the more than two hundred workers who came to Knidos when the dig was operating. Knidos itself exists primarily as an archaeological site, an ancient ruined city. It was once a thriving commercial port and home to the most celebrated statue in antiquity: Praxiteles' nude Aphrodite, now lost, though numerous copies exist.

Iris had told me when we met in New York that we would be setting up tents on the beach facing a small, protected cove, a frequent stopover for yachts traveling the Turquoise Coast. The view from above, near the garrison, was lovely: the curved white beach a crescent, the water clear and blue. But it was empty. The open pavilion where we would eat was deserted. The workrooms were boarded up. The archaeologists were still in Bodrum, the staging area. By then I was exhausted from three straight days of un-air-conditioned travel, sunburned, and suffering the effects of food poisoning.

The commander of the small garrison, young, handsome,

gracious, and probably bored, was delighted to serve as host. For sleeping he could offer only a storeroom with a cot and sacks of supplies (and a window!), but he produced a sumptuous dinner. In his broken English and my smattering of phrasebook Turkish, we chatted on the flat roof together in the evening air, while his underlings brought olives, grilled fish, eggplant, and lamb. At the end of the meal, he produced a large ripe fig, which he tore open with his fingers. The inside was crimson, moist, dotted with small black seeds. Luscious, revolting, alarming, nauseating. It seemed only polite to eat it.

That night I made my way repeatedly down the rocky path to the only available facilities, a toilet that was flushed manually with a bucket of seawater. The runoff went into the cove. Some weeks later, back in Knidos with the archaeological team, we ate an octopus caught in that cove by one of the local boys, who tenderized it by beating it on the rocks. There was a cholera outbreak in Turkey that summer, and this may suggest how it spread. Later I saw people in a yacht flush the head into another pristine cove.

I finally caught up with the group in Bodrum the next day, after hitching a ride with a vacationing French family in their yacht. Bodrum then, as now, was a picturesque fishing village, already attracting celebrities like the rock impresario Ahmet Ertegun, who owned a house there, and his guests. He and Iris were friends. Later that summer Ertegun visited Knidos with Mick and Bianca Jagger and young Jade. We all trailed around after them.

We spent another week in Bodrum as Iris assembled supplies. A horsey athletic woman in her mid-forties, with weathered skin and short sun-bleached blond hair, Iris was a Guggenheim on her mother's side. She was exuberant, adventurous, and rich enough to fulfill her whims. Her usual excavation outfit was a pair of very short shorts and a T-shirt, and sneakers with tennis socks with pom-poms at the back. She was never without her two dachshunds, Phryne and Carlino, and over the next few months was visited by a stream of glamorous friends. Taking visitors around the site, speaking in one of the six languages she knew, she gave a guided tour that was a theatrical presentation, often leaping onto the three-foot podium where the Aphrodite had once stood and illustrating the goddess's pose.

On July 20, 1969, when much of the world was watching Neil Armstrong take his first steps on the moon, she had found the first traces of that circular platform where the Knidian Aphrodite would have stood gazing out toward the island of Kos. Later she found fragments of a statue that may have been part of the missing Aphrodite herself. She diligently reported her finds in the early years in the *American Journal of Archaeology*, but by the time I met her, her interest—and organization—seemed to have waned.

Iris had not completed her doctorate at NYU's Institute of Fine Arts (after changing the subject of her dissertation three times) but had persuaded the Turkish government to give her an excavation permit for a number of years running. Over the weeks I spent at the dig, I came to think that she was an intuitively brilliant archaeologist, but her lack of academic credentials, her record keeping, and a dispute with the British Museum raised doubts among other archaeologists. As a "wealthy amateur," as a colleague put it, she was a throwback to the Society of Dilettanti, which had first excavated at the site in the early nineteenth century.

I had told Iris from the start that I hoped to write about the dig. Later, when the story was about to be published in *The New Yorker*, she was alarmed by the fact-checker's questions. She enlisted her friend Liz Smith, the columnist, to try to stop publication. William Shawn, venerable and reclusive, stood by me, even though I was a first-time contributor. I don't think she ever excavated at Knidos again.

But for now, in August of 1977, after a few days with the group in Bodrum, we traveled back to Knidos in a fishing boat loaded with crates of Montana-brand lunch meat (the Italian version of Spam); tuna fish in ten-pound cans; long, thin Danish hot dogs; Pepsi; toilet paper; tents; sleeping bags; excavation supplies; the eighteen or so volunteer student archaeologists and their gear; and the dachshunds. The boat rode so low in the water, you could trail your hand over the side. We left after dark and arrived at dawn. We set up the tents on the beach, breaking for a lunch of Montana meat and Pepsi, which, along with okra, turned out to be our dietary staples. It was early August, and the temperature was over one hundred. (It had been unofficially measured at 150 degrees Fahrenheit just southeast of Knidos a few weeks before we arrived.) We found shady spots after lunch (the tents were too hot during the day) and slept.

The next five or six weeks I spent on a rocky hillside in the full sun, annotating and categorizing the small Greek and Byzantine artifacts uncovered by the Turkish men who did the digging. The major sites, the rotunda where Aphrodite may once have stood, and the theater were farther down the hillside. I was a site supervisor, along with a young woman named Spencer Boyd. Spencer was in her early twenties, from a wealthy Pittsburgh family who knew Iris. She had spent several summers at the dig. Three Turkish workers— the pickman (the most skilled), the shovel man, and the cart-it-away man—all knew far more than I did. We communicated with them in what they called Tarzanca (Tarzan language).

The pace was desultory. In the late morning Iris would hike up the hill for a look. The workmen would call to one another, "Iris geliyor!" Iris is coming! The sound echoed off the rocky hillside. She had known many of the workmen since she first excavated there, in 1967, and she asked about their families, or friends who had not shown up for work that year. In the early years they called her "Mudur Bey" (Mr. Director). But now, like everyone else, they called her Iris.

Day after day, Spencer and I sat on the hillside, gossiping about Iris and the other volunteers, talking about food and fresh vegetables, how much we wanted a shower (there was almost no fresh water at the site, not to mention electricity), and whether the mail would ever come. Meanwhile, we shuffled through the dusty fragments: shards of painted pottery and heads from tiny figurines that the Turkish diggers were bringing up. A few of the artifacts were ancient Greek; many more were Roman or Byzantine. In the evening we'd take them down to be sorted and categorized.

Despite sunscreen, a hat, and long midday breaks, I had sun poisoning within days, red-speckled arms and legs. Our station was far from the camp, and since my intestinal problems lingered, I ate and drank as little as I could. I came home with 118 pounds on my five-foot-eight-inch frame. My bowels protested well into the following spring.

Did I somehow pick up something on that grueling trip? Did I come home with a virus or parasite that would within months affect my hearing? Or was the potential for hearing loss always there, seizing the advantage when my immune system was compromised? Either explanation seems far-fetched, but so does losing your hearing one spring day, sitting at your desk, working.

One other possible effect—probably even more far-fetched—has haunted me for years. In the early 1980s, I underwent fertility treatments for more than a year without getting pregnant. I had a procedure to clear my fallopian tubes, and in the year and a half after that I got pregnant three times. Each one was an ectopic pregnancy, the embryo lodged in the fallopian tube. Each ended in a surgical termination of the pregnancy.

I wonder if that parasite or virus affected not only my auditory system but also my reproductive system. I'm left with idiopathic—for both.

VOICES: ROSS WANK

It wasn't until he was actually working in the operating room that the physician Ross Wank knew he needed to do something about his hearing. He had gotten successfully through high school, college, medical school, and radiological training with severe hearing loss. But when he needed to relay results of X-rays and CT scans, he finally felt impaired. He couldn't use the telephone, he told me, and would find himself "running around the emergency room to tell people in person, and then running back to go on reading the scans."

The training itself was a challenge. Lectures were often in darkened rooms with slides projected, meaning he could not see the speaker. Working with senior radiologists, he would be looking over their shoulders as they examined a scan, meaning he couldn't read their lips. His hearing loss also made it seem as if he had attitude problems: "I would get reviews of my work when I was on rotation and they would say something about my bedside manner, being aloof. I'd be like, 'What are you talking about?' I got every answer right, every patient diagnosis right, but I wasn't hearing them and I wasn't as involved as I should have been. I would just bow out of a conversation because I lost it."

One sunny Sunday morning I drove out to Syosset, Long Island, to meet Dr. Ross, as he is fondly known. He is a handsome man in his late thirties. He now has a cochlear implant, mostly hidden by his thick dark hair. He was living in a small two-story town house with his wife and twenty-month-old daughter, whose toys had inevitably taken over much of the space. Ross and his wife were looking to buy a house, but for now the town house, not far from where he grew up, fit a young family.

Ross is director of one of the outpatient radiology facilities of North Shore–Long Island Jewish Hospital, a sprawling medical center that has sent out tentacles all over Nassau County. He gives the impression of brash self-confidence, which is somehow also endearing (maybe because, as he later told me, it's only bravado). Already suffering from hearing loss in high school, he refused to get hearing aids. "I thought I was doing well," he told me. "I was smart, and everybody knew it. I was a star athlete, I was getting A minuses, I had a high enough GPA, you know; I got 1400 on my SATs, so I didn't need—I didn't feel like I needed anything. I had a lot of friends."

He went to Williams College, forgoing the possibility of a scholarship for people with hearing loss because he did not want to admit to his loss or to get hearing aids. Eventually he did get them, but not the powerful ones he needed, because he didn't want anyone to see them. As a result, he couldn't hear lectures. But he read and reread the textbook, and usually "aced the test." He got into Mount Sinai School of Medicine and repeated the lecture/textbook process. In lectures, he said, "I would sit there and do the *New York Times* crossword puzzle. I got very good at it." He was accepted into a radiology residency, and that's where his hearing problems caught up with him.

After he finally got an implant (he plans to get a second), Ross became a crusader for implants: "I want to help people with their indecision. I realize I was an idiot for waiting so long to do something about it."

For all his success, he suffered, especially socially. "It affected me meeting girls and having girlfriends. Being made fun of for not hearing things, where people were making light of it. It hurt, but you'd never admit to it. People would say, 'You can hear, you just didn't pay attention.'" And that was partly accurate. "I stopped paying attention because I couldn't hear."

As he told the story of his high school and college years, I'd commented on his resiliency. Late in the conversation, he came back to that. "I don't want you to think I was resilient. It was very, very hard. And I had a lot of bad moments, and a lot of, I wouldn't say depression over it, but it definitely affected me, affected my personality, affected who I became."

He regrets he didn't acknowledge his loss earlier. "Most people are inherently good and inherently sympathetic," he said. "But until you give them a chance—like you, like me, we never gave them a chance . . ." He trailed off. "It's always easier in retrospect, it's easy to tell someone else what to do, but when you're that person, it's always very hard to listen."

THREE

Bring in 'Da Noise!

The sad truth is that many of us are responsible for our own hearing loss. The cause isn't disease or genetics or accidental exposure to a toxin or an explosion. It's the noise we blithely subject ourselves to day after day. Fifteen percent of Americans between the ages of twenty and sixty-nine have noise-induced hearing loss, according to the National Institute on Deafness and Other Communication Disorders (NIDCD). Most won't go as deaf as I did, but many will lose some degree of their hearing. And with that loss, they'll experience disruption, dislocation, a life thrown out of whack. Their families will be frustrated, their colleagues offended or disdainful. They'll feel uncertain, undermined, off-balance but not sure exactly why.

And in most cases it need never have happened. By far the majority of hearing loss in America is noise-related.

In French, the term *"chercher noise à quelqu'un"* means to pick a fight, to look for a quarrel. The term is probably franglais, deriving from the Old English definition of "noise," which also meant "strife" or "quarrel."

The English word itself originates in the French term "nausée"— nausea. For those of us with hearing aids, which seem to amplify indiscriminately, that derivation is apt. A very loud environment can make me feel sick. That's why people with hearing aids take them off or turn them down in restaurants. It's better to hear nothing than too much. We are often also quarrelsome, irritated at the world and at our inability to hear it properly.

The term "noise" is not always negative. "Make a joyful noise unto the Lord," the King James version of the Bible tells us. "Thro' the noises of the night/She floated down to Camelot," Tennyson wrote of his Lady of Shalott. "Beethoven's Fifth Symphony is the most sublime noise that has ever penetrated into the ear of man," E. M. Forster wrote in *Howards End*—ironically perhaps, since the party at the concert proceeds to chatter through the symphony.

What would *Bring in 'Da Noise, Bring in 'Da Funk* have been without the percussive clatter of those tapping feet? Who wants to go to a sports event where the crowd is silent? The excited din of a good party, the bustle and musical sound track of a hip restaurant, the audible energy of a big city, the stomp of a tyrannosaurus in Sensurround, a rock concert in an outdoor amphitheater: noise is an integral part of any of these. *Merriam-Webster's* defines noise as "sound . . . that lacks agreeable musical quality or is noticeably unpleasant." But that is a subjective definition. What's music to my ears is noise to yours.

How loud is too loud? OSHA allows eight hours a day of exposure to 90 decibels, six hours at 92, four hours at 95, two hours at 100, and so on, up to fifteen minutes or less at 115 decibels. The National Institute of Occupational Safety and Health (NIOSH) sets a much higher standard. Its recommendation is for no more than eight hours a day at 85 decibels, two hours at 91 decibels, fifteen minutes at 100, and thirty seconds or less at 115 decibels.

The decibel is calculated according to a logarithmic scale. The threshold of sound is zero decibels. Very few humans can hear at that level. A person with normal hearing begins to hear sound when it reaches 10 or 20 decibels. Each 10-decibel increase represents ten times the loudness and intensity of the previous number. Thus 10 decibels is ten times as loud as 1, though it's still only as loud as a pin dropping. Twenty decibels is one hundred times (ten times ten) as loud as 1 (still very quiet), with the numbers increasing exponentially. A quiet library measures 30 decibels. Normal conversation measures about 60 decibels. A lawn mower measures

90 decibels. The human pain threshold for sound, which varies according to the individual, is about 130 decibels.

• • •

Sports proudly proclaims its decibel levels. We want our stadiums rocking with noise, to cheer on and motivate the athletes (though the athletes themselves sometimes wear earplugs), and to rattle the opposition. The vuvuzelas that characterized the 2010 World Cup in South Africa measured 127 decibels by some counts, 138 by others (a chain saw is 110 decibels). The international soccer organization FIFA rejected calls from other teams to ban the horns. "I have always said that Africa has a different rhythm, a different sound," FIFA president Sepp Blatter said in a Twitter post. "I don't see banning the music traditions of fans in their own country." Masincedane Sport, licensed to manufacture the three-foot plastic horns for the games, blamed counterfeits. The manufacturer's own version met EU levels, a spokesman said, at 113 decibels—that is, louder than a chain saw.

In South Africa, as elsewhere, the noise was all about home court advantage. In 2010, ESPN and Penn State did a study of the loudest college basketball arenas. The University of Kansas's historic Allen Fieldhouse came in first. "Rule No. 1 of home court advantage," the article said. "You need a raucous student section to make a gym shake." Allen Fieldhouse flashes the decibel level on a large screen centered above the court: it can hit 116 decibels before the game even begins. In a review of the 1998–1999 season, *Sports Illustrated* gave top noise billing to the Pit, the University of New Mexico's sunken arena, where in a game against Arizona the decibel level hit 118. (Some bloggers claim it reached 127.) Whether Allen Fieldhouse or the Pit rightfully claims preeminence is a perennial debate.

Noise is an integral part of other spectator sports as well (golf and tennis excepted). At game seven of the 2006 Stanley Cup finals at the RBC Center in Raleigh, North Carolina (which the home-team

Hurricanes won), ESPN measured crowd noise at 138 decibels. Autzen Stadium in Eugene, Oregon, affectionately referred to as "the House of Loud," anecdotally gets the number one spot for loudest college football stadium, with decibel levels as high as 127.2 even though it has a capacity of only 59,000. Michigan Stadium, "The Big House," had a capacity of 106,201 but measured only 100 decibels before renovations began in 2008. Bloggers blamed the fans for not yelling loud enough. When the renovated stadium opened in 2010, capacity had grown to 109,901, but the promise of 30 percent more noise was apparently not met. As one college football blog put it: "What do you get when you amplify silence? How is Michigan Stadium suddenly going to get loud if the fans don't bother making noise?"

One of the loudest domed stadiums (as with all claims to be the loudest, there are disagreements) is the Hubert H. Humphrey Metrodome in Minneapolis: during the second game of the 1987 World Series, between the Minnesota Twins and the St. Louis Cardinals, the decibel level reached 125, comparable to a jet airliner and close to the threshold of pain. The 2010 Super Bowl, played in Miami's Sun Life Stadium, where the New Orleans Saints beat the Indianapolis Colts, is memorable for a photo of one-year-old Baylen Brees, son of the Saints' quarterback, wearing noise-canceling earmuffs, which reduced the stadium noise (over 100 decibels) by 22 decibels.

At Arrowhead Stadium, home of the Kansas City Chiefs, where the crowd noise at a 2003 pre-playoff game was measured at 116 decibels, Chiefs president Carl Peterson said, "I would like to personally challenge our fans—our twelfth man—to push the decibel level at Arrowhead into the 120s."

As for pro basketball, a blogger named Arthur Dobrin fondly remembered games at Madison Square Garden, where he could hear the squeak of the sneakers and the bounce of the ball on the court. You can still hear the squeak and the bounce, but now thanks to the sophisticated noise enhancement systems. The technology involves much more than simply amping up the volume.

"With fans spoiled by earbud fidelity and 5.1-channel home theater systems, owners like the Mavericks' Mark Cuban have turned hosting a game into producing an event—with 'assisted resonance' and 'crowd enhancement,' buzzwords for insiders and euphemisms for others," Alan Schwarz wrote in *The New York Times*. In addition to the sixty speakers hanging over the court, blasting music and other sound effects, microphones in the backboard amplify rim clangs, sneaker squeaks, and, as Schwarz wrote, "the occasional player profanity." The crowd itself is amplified, making it as loud in the mezzanine as in the courtside seats. As he and Mavericks team executive Martin Woodall waited for the start of a game at the American Airlines arena in Dallas, Woodall "whooped gleefully over the din: 'My clothes are shaking.'"

Athletes also like personal sound. MP3 players and headphones are ubiquitous among runners. In 2007, USA Track and Field announced a ban on the use of personal music devices in marathons. Several marathon associations said they wouldn't enforce it, including the New York City Marathon, citing the difficulty of monitoring 38,000 runners wearing postage stamp–size iPod Nanos. In 2008, the USATF lifted the ban, recognizing that marathons have become events not just for elite runners but for the masses—or that subset of the masses that can run twenty-six miles—and that for many recreational runners music helps set their pace and keep them running.

Go into any gym and you'll see sweaty bodies on the treadmill or the rowing machine or the elliptical trainer, pumping away to the private beat of Beyoncé or Rihanna or Jay-Z. The gym itself is a din of pounding feet, grunts and heavy breathing, clanging weights, and sometimes an overlay of pop music, but most of the exercisers are getting their music through earbuds. In a 2008 article in *The Sport Journal*, published by the United States Sports Academy, Costas Karageorghis and David-Lee Priest of Brunel University in London analyzed the effect of music on different levels of exercise. During training, music can result in a 10 percent drop in perceived exertion; it has less effect on high-intensity effort at, say,

85 percent of aerobic capacity, but it still affects the athlete's mood and perception of the effort: "It makes hard training seem like more fun," the authors wrote.

Music also has a physiological effect, with the tempo regulating movement and prolonging performance. The authors cite the Ethiopian marathoner Haile Gebrselassie, who listened to the techno song "Scatman" as he repeatedly broke world records. The tempo, 135 beats per minute, perfectly matched his stride. Too bad for those whose stride it didn't match: he liked it broadcast over the sound system during his races.

Karageorghis, who has been studying the effects of music on physical performance for more than twenty years, suggested a playlist for the casual exerciser: Rihanna's dance remix of "Umbrella," "Push It" by Salt-N-Pepa, "Drop It Like It's Hot" by Snoop Dogg. Weight lifters and bodybuilders prefer heavy metal or hip-hop. Shawn Perine, a senior writer at *Flex* magazine, told *The New York Times* that after a grueling series of squats, LL Cool J's "Mama Said Knock You Out" perks him right up. Bill Conti, who wrote the theme song from *Rocky*, declined to analyze its energizing properties: "Music is anti-intellectual," he told the *Times*. "We know the Greeks went into battle listening to music in the Dorian mode. I can only imagine some Greek guy said, 'This works.'" (You can hear a scale played in the Greek Dorian mode on Wikipedia—unless you have hearing loss, in which case you'll have a hard time distinguishing the notes.) Richard Einhorn, a composer with severe hearing loss, notes that pop music today often uses the Dorian mode, a modified minor scale.

Stage a rock concert in a stadium or sports arena and the sound effects are exponential. Three or four earsplitting concerts may not harm the listener, most people think (Sharon Kujawa and Charles Liberman at Harvard would disagree), but for the musicians the cumulative exposure can lead to permanent hearing problems. Among the many musicians with hearing loss or tinnitus resulting from their performances are Neil Young, Ozzy Osbourne, Will.i.am (who says a painful ringing in his ears drives him to create music at all hours of the day), Jeff Beck, and Eric Clapton. As for The Who, the band that left me with ringing ears for hours after that concert in 1976, every member has suffered hearing impairment. Pete Townshend, who suffers tinnitus as well as hearing loss, describes it as debilitating; it wasn't just the loud music but noise from the pyrotechnics and smashing instruments that punctuated their performances. Their collective hearing problems may have affected their halftime performance at Super Bowl XLIV, which got decidedly mixed reviews: "The Who will always be great, but that was not singing."

There are many contenders for the title of loudest rock band. Among them, chronologically, are Led Zeppelin ("Heartbreaker," 1969, claimed to hit 130 decibels), Deep Purple (the Guinness Book of World Records named them "loudest pop band" after a live 1972 concert), AC/DC, KISS (in 2009, Ottawa authorities forced the band to turn down the sound after it was measured at 136 decibels, 46 decibels over the official festival limit of 90). The heavy metal band Manowar claims to hold the record for a 2008 concert measured at 139 decibels, but the Guinness Book of World Records, in the interest of conserving hearing, has dropped the category of "loudest band."

In many cases, alas, you don't have to be there to hear the noise. A study of the acoustical effects on the surrounding locale of the White River Amphitheatre, a 20,000-seat arena, was presented at the 2011 meeting of the Acoustical Society of America. The stadium, located thirty-five miles southeast of Seattle, is in a hilly rural area, on property owned by the Muckleshoot Indian tribe, reported the researchers Ioana Park and Jeanette Hesedahl of BRC Acoustics and Technology Consulting. Once the basic structure and roof of the amphitheater were completed, two neighboring counties asked for an environmental noise review. It turned out that the sound traveled unevenly, because of geography and the design of the stadium, rather than in concentric circles. Noise mitigation procedures brought the sound down to an acceptable level.

It's not just rock and roll. Classical musicians can be damaged by the music they play. Symphonic music, according to information assembled by Galen Carol Audio, can get as loud as 120 to 137 decibels. Tchaikovsky's *1812 Overture*, often followed by fireworks; Wagner's "Ride of the Valkyries"; the final scene of Puccini's *Turandot*, Richard Strauss's *Also Sprach Zarathustra* with its fanfare, are all very loud pieces of music.

The liner notes to ArkivMusic's album *Earquake—The Loudest Classical Music Of All Time* says of Jón Leifs's *Hekla*, recorded at Finlandia Hall in 1997, "We believe that the final track, 'Hekla,' is probably the loudest single piece of music ever written. It describes, in very graphic terms, 'the eruption of Hekla, Iceland's largest active volcano.' The 140-piece orchestra (which wore earplugs for the recording sessions) includes organ, chorus, and a twenty-two-person percussion section sporting—among other hardware—four sets of rocks hit with hammers, two heavy metal chains, anvils, steel plates, sirens, and several dozen cannon shots." ArkivMusic did not measure the decibel levels, but the liner notes conclude: "DO NOT adjust the volume to comfortable listening levels. If your speakers (and your hearing) aren't in jeopardy, it just isn't an EARQUAKE experience!"

A study published by the Sound Advice Working Group found that the average decibel levels of many orchestral instruments are quite loud. A violin or viola, for instance, can hit a peak of 116 decibels, a flute 118, percussion instruments 123 to 134. These peak levels affect the players themselves as well as those close to them. Peak levels are rarely sustained for a length of time, but musicians put in not only a lot of performing time but even more practice time. The study notes, "Orchestral musicians can reach the upper exposure action value by playing for as little as 10–25 hours per week."

Risk assessment recommendations include having a mixed repertoire of quieter and louder pieces; rehearsing noisy instruments separately from quiet ones; and in a full rehearsal, working only with the players or sections necessary when repeating passages that need correction. Strategic matching of the program to the venue is also important. Mahler's Eighth Symphony, to take an extreme example, not only requires a hall big enough to accommodate a huge orchestra and several choruses, but the right acoustics. (At its premiere in 1910 there were more than a thousand musicians and singers onstage. In February 2012, Gustavo Dudamel conducted 1400 musicians in the so-called Symphony of a Thousand.) Spacing the players adequately, using acoustic panels, and installing risers at various heights all help protect the musicians. Acoustic screens can backfire if not used properly, reflecting the noise back and doubling the noise exposure of the percussionist or trombonist while protecting those in front, and whoever installs them needs to be an expert in acoustics.

• • •

People who go to rock concerts and college or professional sporting events expect noise. But not everyone who goes to a restaurant enjoys an aural assault along with the food. Unless you go to a hushed, old-fashioned, red leather–booth kind of eatery, that may be what you'll get. Restaurants are routinely and deliberately noisy; some of the most expensive are also some of the noisiest.

It starts with the architecture. The trend in restaurants has been large open spaces; walls of windows; high beamed ceilings; wood or tile floors; no curtains or tablecloths; an open kitchen; and two or three hundred diners. "You go to a restaurant, by the time you go home you're exhausted," one researcher, John Carey of Johns Hopkins, told me. A lanky, affable man, he expressed repeated exasperation with unnecessary noise—everywhere from restaurants to background sound effects on NPR. At the start of the interview, he picked up my little tape recorder and announced into it, "This is John Carey, professor of otolaryngology and head and neck surgery." Halfway through the interview, in his enthusiasm for his subject, he accidentally pressed the stop button. (After that, I always made sure the tape recorder sat on the table.)

Open kitchens are popular in home architecture as well. I made the mistake of having one installed when we renovated an old farmhouse. It's beautiful: thirty-foot ceilings, banks of windows overlooking the fields and the barn, a bare hardwood floor. And it's extremely hard for me to hear anyone speak in it.

Open-plan architecture can negatively affect even those who hear well. In an interview in 2003 with *The New York Times*, the *New Yorker* writer Ved Mehta, who is blind, talked about the house on Islesboro, Maine, he had built (he also wrote a book about it). He had given free rein to the architect, Edward Larrabee Barnes. His one request, he said, was for a quiet house, because his spatial clues come from sound. Instead, the article went on, "what he got was a lesson in the acoustic properties of modern building materials like wallboard and glass, which transmit or reflect sound." All clean and angular, with sliding glass doors and mahogany trim, the surfaces bounced sounds harshly around the boxy rooms, and an open staircase carried noise from the basement to the third floor.

"The house is built for the eye, not the ear," Mehta told the *Times*. "Everything in the house was done visually. Modern architects are interested in light and air," he added. "They don't care about sound."

The noise level at restaurants isn't incidental. Restaurants crank up the noise to crank up their profits. Studies have shown that loud, fast music speeds up chewing (and turns tables faster). It also encourages more drinking. A 2008 French study found that turning up the music in a bar resulted in patrons finishing an eight-ounce beer in 11.5 minutes, as opposed to 14.5 minutes at normal sound levels.

Some chefs, as well, like it noisy—cooking to music blasted loud enough to be heard over the clatter of pots and pans. Chef Mario Batali likes Radiohead and Guns N' Roses at Babbo, his flagship New York restaurant, according to *The Wall Street Journal*. Wolfgang Puck prefers Led Zeppelin, Pink Floyd, and The Who at Spago, his celebrity-filled Los Angeles restaurant.

But many patrons (and not just those of a certain age) would rather not eat to the beat of Radiohead. Noise is the second most common complaint about restaurants, according to Zagat, following poor service.

"My hobbyhorse now, because I'm middle-aged," says John Carey, "is that there's a huge ignorance in our society about this issue of background noise. Architects and engineers have no understanding of the tremendous degradation to communication that results from failure to minimize background noise."

When I tell people I'm writing a book about hearing loss and noise, the first thing they say (after telling me that they or their spouse or their mother or friend or cousin also suffers hearing loss) is how noisy restaurants are. They ask for recommendations for places where they might hear each other speak. Or which table in a specific restaurant is going to be most conducive to conversation.

Retailers also pump up the volume. Noise is often part of a store's ambience, as anyone who has ever happened into Urban Outfitters, American Apparel, or the now defunct Virgin Records in Times Square could attest. The adults come out reeling. The kids, the target market, pull out their credit cards.

• • •

Even young children are exposed to excessive levels of noise. The Sight & Hearing Association at the University of Minnesota does an annual survey of toys. In 2004, it found that nine of eleven toys meant for children under five made more than 100 decibels of sound. Among the worst offenders was a "book"—*Barney Songs*—which measured 115 decibels. Home Depot's workman's screwdriver (for kids) was 112. In November 2010, the group's two top offenders were the Bell Riderz Block Blaster bicycle horn and the Fisher-Price Shake 'n Go Ramone toy car, at 129.2 and 119.5, respectively.

That level leads to a risk of hearing damage almost instantly, according to NIOSH. Seven of the eighteen toys meant for children

four and under tested at louder than 100 decibels. Even toys that
might be safe at a distance are usually played with at close range,
the group notes, partly because of children's shorter arm span, partly
because kids just like to hold their toys up close. The group notes
that the Consumer Product Safety Commission does not have regulations about the loudness of toys.

In 2008, a writer who called himself Blogger Dad offered his
own tongue-in-cheek recommendations for children's toys. Of the
perennially popular Fisher-Price Corn Popper, meant for kids one
and up, his "quick rundown" of who should avoid this toy included
"people with ears, parents prone to hangovers, people with pets."
Second on Blogger Dad's list was the Pooh Tick-Tock Clock Activity Choo Choo. The quick rundown: "Who this toy is for: Children
one to three years of age. Deaf parents, children who like loud things,
sadists."

Blogger Dad is less scientific but funnier than Irene Helen
Zundel, who in 2003 noted that among other loud toys, toy
phones for children can be as loud as 129 decibels. Zundel recommends quieter activities like art projects, reading, puzzles, or gar-
dening.

· · ·

Unsurprisingly, New York is loud. In 2010, researchers Richard
Neitzel and Robyn Gershon took decibel-level readings at sixty
public spaces in Manhattan. Ninety percent were chosen based on
the frequency of noise complaints, 10 percent because of their
intrinsic interest—Times Square and Columbus Circle among
them. Measurements were taken at ten-minute intervals between
nine a.m. and five p.m. Monday through Friday, and then were
averaged.

Their conclusions were dispiriting: "Ninety-eight percent of
the noise levels of public spaces in NYC exceeded recommended
community noise levels." The researchers also studied four New
York "pocket parks," havens of quiet in noisy midtown. The pocket

parks—Paley, Greenacre, Tudor City Gardens, and Jackson Square—were far quieter than their surroundings, but still not "quiet." Paley Park, for instance, on East Fifty-third, a lovely small garden with a waterfall, measured 78.9 decibels.

Neitzel and Gershon had earlier studied noise levels in the New York City Transit System, including the subway, much of which was built more than one hundred years ago. Using a complicated series of measurements, they found that nearly one in five subway stations (combining platform noise and noise of the train) exceeded 85 decibels. The authors also found that subway noise in 2007, the year they did their measurements, was lower than in earlier studies. A 1931 study found sound levels ranging from 87 to 97 decibels. A 1971 study found levels that ranged from 87 to 110, with the highest levels on Queens and Manhattan lines, both at the platform level and inside cars. The authors attribute these earlier high decibel levels to "possible differences in measurement equipment and protocols."

Maybe. But any New Yorker who has ridden the subway over the past forty years can tell you that in 1971 the subway was much louder than it is today. Subway cars were not air-conditioned, the windows were open much of the time, and the equipment in general—the construction of the cars, the wheels on the tracks, the warning signals and horns, the announcements in the trains and stations—was considerably louder than it is today. I still remember the earsplitting screech of the 4 train on a hot summer day, the windows open, negotiating the sharp curve going south into Grand Central Station. The authors also failed to take into consideration that until the Sony Walkman came on the market in 1979, boom boxes were common on trains, despite signs that prohibited radio playing (along with spitting and smoking).

The toll of all this noise on human health goes beyond damage to hearing, Neitzel and Gershon noted. "Excessive noise exposure may be linked to hypertension and ischemic heart disease, disruptions in stress hormones, and sleep disorders." Not to mention the "adverse social, psychological, and occupational effects associated with" irreversible noise-induced hearing loss.

I occasionally take my decibel-level reader (originally the Pyle PSPL01 Mini Digital, though I now use an iPhone app called sound-AMP R) around the city with me. The Pyle measures from 40 to 130 decibels, using C-type frequency weighting instead of the A-type used by professionals, a technicality that seemed irrelevant for my uses. It claims accuracy within 3.5 decibels and seems responsive to minimal changes in sound.

At home in my apartment, the noise level averages 50 to 55 decibels, thanks to carpeting and cozy furniture, and a view over backyards rather than the street. My block, West Ninetieth between West End Avenue and Riverside Drive, averages 72 to 78 decibels if there is no traffic, construction, or garbage trucks. The IRT platform at Ninety-sixth Street and Broadway with a train coming into the station: 90 to 96. On the 2 express train, windows closed, the measurement is 92 to 107. On an uncrowded R train, 90 to 92—loud enough to drown out an announcement that sounded like "Take three Excedrin." A nearly empty Pret A Manger near Union Square, mid-afternoon, 78 to 80. A Union Square subway platform for the BMT, 90 to 92.

These are relatively quiet environments—relative, that is, to the rest of the city. I did not go to midtown. I didn't travel in rush hour. There were no panhandlers, drummers, Mexican mariachi players, or boys break-dancing on the subway. I didn't encounter a fire engine or ambulance. I was not on a subway car with sixty shrieking fourth-graders. At home, I didn't run the blender or the food processor. No one was using a leaf blower or lawn mower. I didn't see any garbage trucks. Nobody shot a gun (160–170 decibels, according to the Center for Hearing and Communication). It wasn't the Fourth of July (fireworks measure 162 decibels three feet from the explosion, which is still pretty loud on the ground).

Subway conductors routinely wear noise-canceling headphones. People operating jackhammers often do, but the people working around them often don't. Anyone on the flight deck of an aircraft carrier (150 decibels) wears hearing protection. It's so loud that even radio communication is impossible, so the crews communicate nonverbally. If you happened to be 161 kilometers from Krakatoa when it exploded, according to calculations based on barometric measurements, the noise level was 180 decibels. The call of the blue whale, the largest and loudest animal on earth, measures about 188 decibels.

. . .

Is it noisier now than it used to be?

Dickens's London was notoriously noisy. He described the street musicians as "brazen performers on brazen instruments, beaters of drums, grinders of organs, bangers of banjos, clashers of cymbals, worriers of fiddles, and bellowers of ballads." The street musicians had a lot of competition: the clatter of carriage wheels on cobblestone streets, street vendors hawking their wares, the shouts of newsboys and cabbies, the barking of London's numerous dogs, warning bells clanging, the bustle of hundreds of busy people, shoes and boots tap-tapping, and the clip-clopping of horses.

The death of John Leech, Dickens's friend and the illustrator of *A Christmas Carol*, was attributed to the aggravation of London's street noise, especially its street musicians. Noise worsened his heart condition and his delicate nerves. His final words to fellow artist William Powell Frith indicate the depth of his misery: "Rather, Frith, than continue to be tormented in this way, I would prefer to go to the grave where there is no noise." Days later Leech got his wish, bringing him the quiet he felt he had been unjustly denied in life.

One scholar estimated that there were more than a thousand organ-grinders in London in mid-century, many of them reflecting London's new immigrant underclass. Antipathy settled on Italian organ-grinders. A writer for the *City Press* commented that the musicians were "as filthy in speech as in looks . . . They howl like so many apes and baboons escaped from the Zoological Gardens." The writer went on: "No Londoner should sally forth to business without first spiking, or hanging, or shooting one of the howlers of the streets."

Dickens's contemporary Thomas Carlyle grew more and more impatient with the noise on Cheyne Row the longer he lived there, and in 1853 his patience gave out: Referring to himself as "the UNPROTECTED MALE," he wrote a bloodthirsty screed: "Those Cocks must either withdraw or die." He reserved special venom for a "vile yellow Italian" organ-grinder: "The question arises, Whether to go out and, if not assassinate him, call the Police upon him, or to take myself away to the bath-tub and the other side of the house?"

Instead, he built himself a soundproof study (the construction noise nearly drove him over the edge), with double-thick walls, insulated skylights, and a specially designed slate roof with sound-deadening air chambers underneath. But something went wrong. The result, George Prochnik writes, was "a fiasco." The soundproof study had somehow ended up being the noisiest room in the house. Carlyle was convinced the builder had deceived him. In despair over the venality of human nature, not to mention the expense and shoddy results, he shut himself in a stovepipe. Fortunately, a maid found him before he was overcome by the fumes.

The Metropolitan Police Act passed in 1839 greatly expanded the city police force and empowered them to make arrests against all sorts of public nuisances, including "furious driving," selling pornography on the street, and "wantonly disturbing people" by ringing doorbells. It stopped short in its powers to control street musicians, merely mandating that they must move on when asked.

New York was encouraged to pass a similar law against the raucous noise created by newsboys, where the same anti-immigrant undertone sullied the calls for tranquillity. In New York in the early part of the twentieth century, a New York resident, quoted in David Nasaw's *Children of the City*, wrote that the boys were "an unmitigated nuisance in the neighborhoods they invade," as well as a health hazard for those who were "sick or nervous . . . Doctors will testify that the chances of recovery for their patients are sometimes seriously impaired by the raucous shouts portentous of calamity."

The shouting of newsboys or the incessant and often off-key tunes of organ-grinders, even the cymbal clashers (unless you spent too much time near one, or were a cymbal clasher yourself), seem quaint compared to a steel drum in the subway station or a Harley revving up or the neighbor using a leaf blower under your bedroom window.

New York is the noisiest city in the world, according to the World Health Organization (WHO). The average decibel level on a midtown street is 90. The next noisiest cities, in order, are Tokyo, Nagasaki, Buenos Aires, Mumbai, Delhi, Calcutta, and Madrid. In hot high-density cities like Buenos Aires and Calcutta, the noise is loud even indoors, especially in poor areas without air-conditioning. In colder climates, closed windows act as a barrier.

The result of all that noise is hearing loss, the most frequently occurring sensory deficit in developing countries. WHO estimated in 2010 that more than 275 million people around the world suffered from hearing impairment. Adult-onset hearing loss, it stated, was the second-leading cause of disability. And the organization left no doubt that the primary cause is noise, with the significance of other possible causes—ear infections, for instance—thought to be "negligible."

· · ·

And what about those ubiquitous iPods? Two recent studies published within months of each other, both by Harvard scientists, both using the National Health and Nutrition Examination Survey, found two completely different trends. The first: "The prevalence of any hearing loss increased significantly from 14.9 percent to 19.5 percent" in teenagers over the past decade. The second found no change. Common sense would tell you that any teenager listening to his iPod loud enough for his parents to hear it, for eight or ten hours a day, is damaging his hearing. The only takeaway I found from these two studies is another example of how statistics can mislead. I discuss these studies at greater length in the Notes, pages 252–253.

No matter what the true story is about today's teenagers, the aging of the baby boomer generation means that more and more of us will be affected by natural hearing loss associated with aging. If there's not an epidemic now—and the conflicting statistics about teenagers leave that an open question—there may well be one in the near future.

We're the generation that grew up with Pink Floyd and the Rolling Stones, went to concerts at Madison Square Garden and the Meadowlands, fought in Vietnam. We were the Walkman generation (much louder than iPods are today, with no noise cap). We went to earsplitting concerts, ate in restaurants where we couldn't hear ourselves talk, shouted ourselves hoarse at sporting events. No one ever thought of turning down the noise.

VOICES: JACQUI METZGER

It's hard to think of a profession less amenable to hearing loss than psychoanalysis. The patient lies on the couch, facing away from the analyst, meaning he or she cannot read the patient's lips. Every word in analysis is important, and sometimes the most important are mumbled or hinted at and then dropped. It takes an acute ear to pick up on those clues and press the patient to follow through on those thoughts.

Jacqui Metzger, a psychoanalyst in Seattle, has continued to practice through years of deafness, thanks to technology. We met at her office, in a low-slung wood and stone structure in the University of Washington neighborhood, where her colleagues practice psychotherapy and psychoanalysis. She was an attractive woman in her early sixties wearing comfortable Eileen Fisher–style clothes, her office layout that of therapists anywhere: a therapist's chair, a patient's chair facing it, an analyst's couch, her desk. She offered me the therapist's chair since the light would then be behind me instead of behind her, making it easier for me to lip-read. I'd never sat in the analyst's chair and was not only grateful for her thoughtfulness but also got a little thrill out of sitting on that side of the equation.

Her hearing loss was hereditary and progressive and first manifested itself at age six. By the time she was in junior high, she wore two hearing aids. "My hearing loss affected me significantly in all kinds of ways, growing up, and of course it continues to do so now. Back then it wasn't something anybody really talked about; you just pulled yourself up by your bootstraps and paid attention. In college I sat in the front row in my classes, and managed to make my way through." After college she taught skiing, and then, when she was twenty-eight, she decided it was time to think about "real" work.

She got a master's degree in deafness rehabilitation at NYU, began to learn sign language, and worked with deaf and deaf-blind people in New York. She moved to Seattle and got her M.S.W. at the University of Washington. She was the first deaf student in the program and remembers having to write to the president of the university requesting interpreter services. Now there is a full-time and very busy Coordinator of Interpreter Services at UW.

She received her first cochlear implant fourteen years ago, which improved her hearing significantly, and a few years later she embarked on a program of psychoanalytic training. Her own training analysis was "extraordinarily helpful in understanding myself not only as a person but as a person with hearing loss, and the impact that hearing loss had on me and who I am now."

Although most of her patients do not have hearing loss, she specializes in working with people who are deaf or hard of hearing. "I met a new patient, and after seeing this person a couple of times and feeling somewhat perplexed about our interaction, I said, 'I have this sense we're somehow missing each other as we talk. I wonder if you have a hearing loss.' This person was surprised but said yes, that was true. We talked, and over time we came to understand that not wearing hearing aids was a way of keeping people at a distance, which also had happened in my office with me. Now my patient has a second set of hearing aids, and has discovered satisfaction in closer relationships with other people, and no longer needs to use hearing loss as protection."

I told Metzger how difficult it was to acknowledge hearing loss at the *Times*. "This reminds me of working with hard-of-hearing patients employed at large companies in this area," she said. Seattle is home to Microsoft and Amazon and other technology companies, which, like the *Times*, are competitive and youth oriented. "They felt they couldn't let anybody know, it's just too competitive, they can't ask people to speak more slowly. They assumed if they were to acknowledge their problem, they'd be left behind . . . considered inferior, incompetent." She went on, "The law now protects us, supposedly. The guidelines are all really reasonable. The challenge is advocating for ourselves, and asking for what we need to be productive and competitive."

As for the notion that the person with hearing loss may eventually reach the stage of "acceptance," she demurs: "Acknowledgment, maybe," she said. "Acknowledgment that it's there and not going to go away, and it's real, and that you have to deal with relentless challenges. I think that developing the ability to manage these challenges signifies that someone has come to some kind of peace with it, but you don't really come to accept it fully."

In her tranquil office, looking out on the damp, lush green Seattle courtyard, she seemed at peace with herself. But, she added, grief and anger don't go away. They just recede, occasionally to flare up.

FOUR

You Can't See It, but I Can't Hear You

Hearing loss is an invisible disability. There's no white cane to signal a problem, no crutches, no twitches or jerky movements, no bandages or braces. If you have been a hearing person most of your life, you probably talk normally. Most people with hearing loss quickly learn to nod or smile or respond in a noncommittal way, taking their signal from the speaker and the people around them. How many times have I laughed at a joke I didn't hear? How many times have I said, "I'm so sorry," when I had no idea what I was sorry about? How many times have I nodded in agreement to a point I hadn't heard and may not even have agreed with?

Being a person with hearing loss is like being in Paris and knowing just enough French to ask an articulate question, and then being completely unable to comprehend the answer.

Pitfalls, snafus, glitches, and potholes mark the conversational path of a person with hearing loss. The trouble is that sometimes you don't even know when you've stepped into one. I've long since stopped participating in group conversations except with my closest friends. I lose the train of the discussion and ask a question that was just answered. I think we're talking about one thing when we're talking about something completely different. We've left that subject already, or maybe we were never discussing it at all. I get bits and pieces, and if the subject is familiar enough I can patch them together. But I dodge anything controversial. Or anyone intimidating.

Since I'm also very good at faking it, many people don't know I'm a person with hearing loss. Instead, they think I'm arrogant or remote, absentminded or distracted, drunk or just plain stupid.

Even when I do understand what is being said, the effort of trying to hear eclipses my ability to think. My brain is so preoccupied with translating the sounds into words that it seems to have no processing power left over to dig into the storerooms of memory for a response. Nor does it have the processing power to tuck away new information—like someone's name.

Frank Lin of Hopkins discussed this phenomenon in more scientific terms in a paper titled "Hearing Loss and Incident Dementia" published in 2011 in the *Archives of Neurology*. "The potential effect of hearing loss on cognitive reserve is suggested by studies demonstrating that, under certain conditions, in which auditory perception is difficult (i.e., hearing loss), greater cognitive resources are dedicated to auditory perceptual processing to the detriment of other cognitive processes such as working memory." Lin noted an increasingly strong correlation between hearing loss and dementia—the greater the hearing loss, the higher the likelihood of dementia. "This reallocation of neural resources to auditory processing could deplete the cognitive reserve available to other cognitive processes," he wrote, "and possibly lead to the early clinical expression of dementia."

Lin's was a prospective study, following 639 individuals aged thirty-six to ninety who were part of the Baltimore Longitudinal Study of Aging. None of the participants had cognitive impairment, as measured in standard tests, at the beginning of the study. Some had hearing loss. The study followed the participants over eighteen years. In an interview in Baltimore shortly after the study was published, Lin amplified on the care taken in the study: "Controlling for age, medical risk factors, diabetes, hypertension, we found that people who began with hearing loss had a greater incidence of dementia." The diagnosis of dementia adhered to the criteria established by the National Institute of Neurological Disorders and Stroke.

How might hearing loss and dementia be related? There are some logical explanations. Hearing loss often leads to social isolation, and social isolation is a risk factor for dementia. The cognitive overload theory is another possible explanation. The third is that there is some common cause, "some pathological process," Lin said, which causes both hearing loss and dementia. For someone like me, this last hypothesis is deeply distressing.

Dementia was associated with mild to moderate hearing loss, but the risk of dementia increased with the degree of hearing loss. The use of hearing aids seemed to have no effect ("Self-reported hearing aid use was not associated with a significant reduction in dementia risk," the study states), but how hearing aids were used was not studied: how long the participant had worn a hearing aid, how often, what type of hearing aid. The paper pointed out the necessity for further study on "whether hearing devices and aural rehabilitation strategies could affect cognitive decline." So far, the effect remains unknown.

"Could we do something to delay the onset of dementia?" Lin asked rhetorically. His voice was tinged with frustration. "It's hugely important, because by 2050 one in thirty Americans will have dementia. If we could delay the onset by even one year, the prevalence of dementia drops by fifteen percent down the road. You're talking about billions of dollars in health care savings."

The Baltimore Longitudinal Study of Aging consisted of a volunteer cohort of individuals of high socioeconomic status, as Lin noted, urging caution about his generalizing from his findings. But since hearing loss occurs in greater numbers in those of low socioeconomic status, as does dementia, it stands to reason that these findings are likely to be conservative when applied to the population as a whole.

. . .

The stigma of deafness dates back to at least 1000 B.C., when Hebrew law granted the deaf limited rights to property and marriage but prohibited them from participating fully in the rituals of the Temple. There are few mentions of the deaf in the Old Testament, but the Danish historian Regi Theodor Enerstvedt cites passages like Leviticus 19:14 as examples of a relatively benign attitude: "Thou shalt not curse the deaf, nor put a stumbling block before the blind."

The ancient Greeks shunned the deaf. Aristotle, in 355 B.C., declared, "Those who are born deaf all become senseless and incapable of reason." Because the deaf could not learn Greek, he said, they were "Barbarians," the ancient Greek term for anyone who was not Greek.

With the early Christians, attitudes toward the deaf became more inclusive. Saint Augustine (A.D. 354–430) wrote that although deafness could be a hindrance to faith, the deaf could learn and therefore were able to receive faith and salvation. He is one of the first to refer to the use of some kind of sign language among the deaf. According to a time line compiled by historians at Gallaudet University in Washington, D.C., "Augustine refers to bodily movements, signs, and gestures" as a means of transmitting thought and belief.

Nevertheless, the New Testament has long been problematic for the deaf. One passage in particular, Mark 9:25, led some to equate deafness with possession by the devil. Jesus meets a child who "foameth, and gnasheth with his teeth, and pineth away." The child is also deaf and cannot speak. "Thou dumb and deaf spirit," Jesus says, "I charge thee, come out of him and enter no more into him."

Fundamentalist Christians still discuss the passage in terms of possession by the devil. Among the most destructive interpretations is that of an evangelist minister, Todd Bentley, author of *The Revelation of the Deaf and Dumb Spirit*. In his ministry, he writes, he does not pray for them to hear, but instead "command[s] the devil that made them deaf to come out of their ears." At first, he wrote, he was able to heal only about 2 percent of the people at his meetings. But when he began exorcising the devil from his parishioners' ears, he said 75 to 80 percent were cured. "I thought, 'hallelujah!'" he wrote.

Bentley is no model of behavior and has been censured by his own church. Convicted of sexual assault as a teenager (he has admitted to being part of a sexual assault ring), he was a substance abuser before his conversion to Christ in his late teens. In 2008, he was kicked out of his Christian ministry, divorcing his wife and marrying the intern he had been having an affair with.

He blames his wayward youth on his mother's deafness. It was her deafness that drove him to a criminal rage as a young teenager, he writes, but also inspired him to focus in his ministry on the deaf. He was unable to cure his mother, he says, but has had more success with others. "One day the Lord Jesus spoke to my heart about the deaf spirit," he writes. "About the boy in the gospels that was deaf and mute. He was possessed with a spirit, but he was deaf and mute. And when Jesus commanded the spirit to come out of the boy, he both heard and spoke. I said, 'That is the key.'"

Why would the devil want to render someone deaf? What's in it for him? Bentley explains: "Do you think the devil wants you to hear the voice of God?"

• • •

The biggest stigma associated with hearing loss is age. Even the hearing aid companies play into this stereotype. Hearing aid ads look a lot like ads for erectile dysfunction—handsome, happy people with gray hair. A brochure for Widex (one of the major hearing aid manufacturers) features an attractive couple, their arms around each other. The man, with crinkly smiling eyes, beautiful teeth, and a sexy stubble, is presumably the hearing aid wearer. There's a hint of a hearing aid behind his ear.

Almost every hearing aid company takes pains to describe its products as "invisible," often including photographs that show the hearing aid just barely detectable in or behind the ear. "The problem with extolling this possibility," wrote Mark Ross, a longtime columnist for *Hearing Loss Magazine,* "is that it simply reinforces the notion that one has some sort of shameful condition that has to be hidden. In other words, the message being conveyed is that the hearing loss itself is a stigma, no matter how invisible the hearing aid."

• • •

It is perhaps because of these stigmas that deafness can be made fun of with so little compunction. Victor Hugo added comic relief to *The Hunchback of Notre Dame* with a scene where the deaf and dumb Quasimodo is brought before a magistrate, who is himself deaf but doesn't admit it, since, as Hugo writes, it was better to be seen as an "imbecile than deaf."

It's nearly unthinkable these days to make fun of people with severe vision problems (Mr. Magoo excepted), or with physical or mental disabilities. Obesity jokes are tasteless. But deafness is still fair game. And as even I must admit, it is often funny.

The British novelist David Lodge began to lose his hearing in his forties and, like many, refused at first to acknowledge it. In his astute and funny novel *Deaf Sentence,* he describes with painful and hilarious accuracy the experience. In the opening paragraph, his protagonist is at a noisy party, trying to hear a woman in a red silk blouse. "For the man now almost nuzzling the bosom of the woman in the red blouse, as he brings his right ear closer to her mouth, the noise reached some time ago a level that makes it impossible for him to hear more than the odd word." Did she say "flight from hell" or was it "cry for help"? They have been talking for ten minutes, and "strive as he may he cannot identify the conversational topic."

Later he notes, "Deafness is comic, as blindness is tragic. Take Oedipus, for instance: suppose, instead of putting out his eyes, he had punctured his eardrums. It would have been far more logical actually, since it was through his ears that he learned the dreadful truth about his past, but it wouldn't have the same cathartic effect."

• • •

The nineteenth-century feminist Harriet Martineau was widely regarded as an opinionated, outspoken old maid. She nevertheless charmed Charles Darwin—who went to pay a "duty call"—with her "agreeable" intelligence. He was also, as he wrote in a letter, "astonished to find out how little ugly she is." Martineau intimidated many visitors with her demands that they speak up, but her own writing betrays her suffering: people with hearing loss, she wrote, "rarely received adequate, or even intelligent, sympathy."

Some turn deafness to a positive. Thomas Edison's hearing loss resulted in his becoming a telegraph operator, which led to his future discoveries. Alexander Graham Bell's mother was deaf, which inspired his study of acoustics. The journalist I. F. Stone's hearing loss, his biographer D. D. Guttenplan wrote, "actually worked to his advantage: His inability to hear the proceedings meant he didn't bother attending the daily round of news briefings," freeing him to "ferret out the nuggets of inconvenient truth."

Joseph Medill, the scion of the Chicago newspaper family, had lost much of his hearing by his early forties, "necessitating a black ear trumpet and dramatically increasing the impression of age," writes Megan McKinney in *The Magnificent Medills*. "Joseph's deafness was selective; it allowed him to screen out the chatter of bores and lightweights while enabling him to carry on one-sided exchanges consisting chiefly of questions and monologues." "It's good to be the king," Mel Brooks's Louis XVI chortles (until his head is chopped off) in *History of the World: Part I*. It is easier to be hard of hearing if you're the boss. But it must still be painful. The isolation and despair—the irritability, depression, impatience, and shame— afflict even the powerful.

And the meek as well. Recently someone commented to me that so-and-so, a mutual friend, was boring, that she never had anything to say and often just sat there, smiling sweetly. I happen to know that this person has a serious hearing loss. I don't know if she has hearing aids, but I do know she can't hear. And I also now know that she's in the early stages of Alzheimer's. As Lin's study showed, my friend's hearing loss and the onset of Alzheimer's may not be a coincidence.

• • •

The loss of any of the five senses is devastating. Most people take their senses—sight, smell, hearing, touch, taste—for granted. You can mimic blindness. All you have to do is blindfold yourself and try to get around. Some people temporarily lose smell or taste when they have a respiratory illness. Hands or feet or toes can become numb for a time and lose all sense of feeling. Hearing can temporarily go after a loud concert. But the permanent loss of a sense is almost impossible to imagine.

Complete and permanent loss of touch is rare, except in isolated neuropathies, but a 2006 article described two individuals who had entirely lost their sense of touch, though not their motor skills. The author described the arduous training that one, Ian Waterman, went through to teach himself to use vision to compensate for the loss of the sense of touch. To perform an action he had to "visually track the state of his body and environment, and exert an extensive, conscious effort to apply appropriate muscle force during the right duration to accomplish the task at hand." He told the author that it was like running a marathon every day.

Waterman needed constant visual feedback to know where his body was in space. If the lights went out suddenly when he was standing up, the author wrote, "Waterman immediately fell to the floor. This was because of his inability to supervise his body without sight."

Loss of taste is a relatively common disorder, though often loss of smell is the true culprit. According to the NIDCD, 200,000 people a year visit doctors for taste disorders. Rarely, a condition called ageusia causes a person to lose all sense of taste. More often, taste disorders include phantom taste perception (tasting something that isn't there) or reduced ability to taste. There can be health consequences. People with diabetes or high blood pressure may use too much sugar or salt because they can't gauge by taste how much they're using. Loss of taste can also lead to depression, according to the NIDCD. (I think the loss of any sense can contribute to depression.) Occasionally the loss of taste is a symptom of a central nervous system disorder, like Parkinson's or Alzheimer's.

The celebrated chef Grant Achatz, of Chicago's Alinea restaurant, told the story of what happened to his career after he developed a life-threatening squamous cell carcinoma on his tongue. A brutal regime of chemotherapy and radiation saved his life (and his tongue). He rarely missed a day of work; he simply trained his chefs to mimic his palate, and he learned to cook using his other senses instead. Eventually he regained his ability to taste, one sensation— sweet, salty, bitter, sour—at a time.

"Smell is the stepchild of the senses, the one that many think they could do without," wrote Robin Marantz Henig, who lost her sense of smell after a fall. "But when I couldn't smell things, I couldn't fully inhabit the world, and my movements in it were somehow, almost imperceptibly, more clumsy."

Henig trained herself to regain her sense of smell. "The first time I smelled cut grass again," she wrote, "in the small park near the American Museum of Natural History, was almost exactly two years after my fall. It made me cry. The tears embarrassed me, but cut grass is one of those fragrances, like my father's oil paints or my mother's L'Air du Temps, that transport me directly to the landscape of childhood. And that's what I had been missing, really, and why getting back my sense of smell was so precious: a visceral connection to the person I used to be."

For the adult with late-onset hearing loss, there is no recovering the person you used to be. You can learn to hear again, but you can never be the hearing person you once were. Even the best devices are a poor substitute for nature's creation.

Losing your hearing is something quite different from losing any other sense. "I have made the bleak journey from the world of hearing to the world of silence," wrote Jack Ashley, a British MP with high expectations of political advancement. He lost his hearing after a viral infection at age forty-five and became profoundly deaf. In a collection of pieces titled *Adjustment to Adult Hearing Loss*, he wrote, "The born deaf are denied the advantages [of the formerly hearing] but they are spared the desolating sense of loss." He went on to be reelected after his hearing loss, and became a strong advocate for people with disabilities.

Going deaf as a child can usually be accommodated to. But going deaf as an adult destroys your world, disables your life. "These individuals have developed a personality that does not incorporate hearing loss," Mary Kaland and Kate Salvatore wrote in *The ASHA Leader*. "They have jobs, families, and personalities and relate to those aspects as fixed." Sylvia in *Tribes* argues with her boyfriend, Billy, who was born deaf in a hearing family. "I know what it's like being deaf!" Billy says. Sylvia retorts: "But you don't know what it's like *going* deaf! I just keep thinking, 'Am I different?' Am I turning into somebody different? I'm becoming a miserable person. I feel like I'm losing my personality . . . I feel stupid."

Or, more formally, as Kaland and Salvatore put it: "Late-deafened adults report that their hearing loss robs them of an understanding of their identity and often initiates an identity crisis." They suffer, as Jack Ashley said, a desolating sense of loss.

• • •

But it need not be only desolating. Much depends on the resiliency and personality of the person with new hearing loss. The artist David Hockney, shortly after he lost much of his hearing in his mid-fifties, was asked by a *New York Times* reporter if he found that his other senses sharpened to compensate. "I once discussed that with somebody," he answered. "I pointed out that if you lose your sight you then use sound to locate yourself in space. Whereas, if you can't locate yourself with sound you probably do sharpen the visual thing."

Hockney's work at the time (1993) included designing sets for operas. A filmmaker who recorded the process later told an interviewer: "He spent up to a year designing each opera. He listened to the opera while he drove through some incredible landscapes, like the Grand Canyon. He listened to the music over and over before he even began to design. This process led to these incredibly intense set designs." She went on, "When he could no longer hear the music well enough, he stopped creating opera sets. However, he continued to paint without restraint. He creates and lives a life full of passion."

Hockney took the *Times* interviewer, Trip Gabriel, on a drive up the Pacific Coast Highway, his stereo blaring loud enough for him to hear it. As Gabriel described it:

> Turning east he climbed through hills sloping like a woman's shoulders as the music segued into the "Blue Danube" waltz. As the Santa Monica Mountains became more rugged, the lilting strains of Strauss gave way, with Mr. Hockney's fingers dancing over the buttons, to mythically stirring Wagner.
>
> He dropped into a valley and entered Malibu Creek State Park. The lovely landscape of live oaks and bald rock outcroppings was reminiscent of northern Spain. Now, the music was an orchestral passage from *Parsifal*, which is, coincidentally, set in the mountainous terrain of that region. Earlier, he had said he was thinking of designing sets for a future *Parsifal* for the Los Angeles Opera. He thought of Wagner's opera, which tells of a king tortured by a spear wound that will not heal, as a meditation on the era of AIDS.

Hockney had lost many friends to AIDS, and now he had lost his hearing. Still, he told Gabriel, "sometimes it baffles me: why don't people just look at the world and see how beautiful it is?"

VOICES: TONI IACOLUCCI

Six years ago, over a period of a week, Toni Iacolucci lost all the hearing in her left ear, a "terrifying" experience, she said. She suffered tinnitus so loud that she wasn't sure she could live with it. She was hospitalized for a week, and given high doses of steroids—to no avail. When she left the hospital, she was profoundly deaf. We met for an interview in the spring of 2012 in my apartment. She read my lips, or read questions that I typed on my computer.

Her hearing loss began in childhood, isolating her to some extent but not seriously enough to require hearing aids. "Often I felt like I was on the outside looking in," she said of her childhood. As an adult, she trained and worked for several years as a social worker, ignoring her increasing hearing loss. After noticing how often her colleagues said she hadn't heard what they said, she went to an audiologist. Actually, she said, she went to three or four audiologists, "looking for someone who could 'cure' me."

She did get a hearing aid at that point, in her left ear, but she was "enormously embarrassed and ashamed to have anyone see it." In her early forties she suddenly lost much of the hearing in her good ear, the right, and a decade later, in her fifties, she had lost enough hearing in the left ear that she was referred for screening for a cochlear implant. Part of the screening was an MRI, which revealed an acoustic neuroma, ruling out the possibility of an implant.

At that point, she had no hearing in the right ear and impaired hearing in the left (with the hearing aid). And then she lost the hearing in that ear too, leaving her profoundly deaf in both ears.

Iacolucci had long since given up social work. For a while she managed restaurants and dance companies, and was co-owner of an "event decor" business. "I always struggled, though, never realizing how much stress and exhaustion my hearing loss was causing." Her friends gathered round when she was hospitalized, and at last she realized that although she had lost her hearing, she was essentially the same person.

The hospital "acted as a transition from my old life as someone with hearing loss to my new life as someone who is deaf," she said. "I experienced a strange sense of euphoria. From the moment we're told we have hearing loss, I think consciously or unconsciously we all fear deafness. But here I was . . . walking, sleeping, eating, hanging out with friends. I'd 'survived' deafness."

After she left the hospital, she set about to amend her driver's license to acknowledge her disability. It took her thirteen hours to finally get the relevant information from the DMV. "Something 'clicked,' with that," she said. "I felt it was unconscionable that anyone should have to go through this, especially since deafness was quite enough to deal with. I spent the next several months e-mailing with the DMV, finally getting them to include the info on their website . . . and I was hooked." What she was hooked on was advocacy.

She served on the planning committee of the New York chapter of the HLAA. (Meetings are live-captioned using CART—Communication Access Realtime Translation—simultaneous captioning.) She designed and wrote the chapter's website and has been very active in Walk4Hearing as a team coordinator and co-chair. In 2011, Walk4Hearing raised $170,000 and drew twelve hundred participants. Her work now, she says, is focused on raising awareness, advocating for CART accessibility, and helping people acknowledge their loss and "feel comfortable" about it.

FIVE

Am I Deaf or Just Dumb?

I was at Penn Station recently to get a train to Washington. The self-service kiosks all had long lines and I was late, so I got in the shorter line to get my ticket from the agent. First she chastised me for coming before she was ready (even though her light had just signaled that her booth was open). Then she grumpily mumbled some questions. I gave her my reservation printout and finally realized she also wanted my driver's license.

When I asked what platform the train was on (it was leaving in five minutes), she made a vague gesture to my left and said something incomprehensible. I had told her I was hard of hearing, I had done what you're supposed to do. But, as happens all too often, she seemed not to comprehend that the healthy-looking, well-spoken person standing on the other side of her glass partition could not hear a word she said. I stumbled off in the direction she'd indicated, embarrassed, furious, and stressed, which only makes my hearing worse, my head spin, my confidence flounder.

I ignored my hearing loss for the first twenty years, existing in a relatively stable state of denial. Then, when it could no longer be ignored, I spiraled into depression, came close to breaking up my marriage, isolated myself from friends, lost my job. Many people with midlife, mid-career hearing loss go through the same cycle of denial, bargaining, anger, depression, and—with the help of audiologists and hearing specialists, and a good psychotherapist— acceptance, or something like it.

Acceptance is elusive, however, shadowed by the anger and shame you've tried so hard to overcome. It doesn't take a lot for anger to get the upper hand.

• • •

The capital-*D* Deaf community these days is vibrant and supportive, with its own language, architecture, and accomplished professionals. There are Deaf lawyers, Deaf surgeons, Deaf actors, and Deaf people in just about every profession. People with hearing loss, by contrast, live in a kind of limbo, not really part of the hearing world but not part of the Deaf world either. Many are unwilling to acknowledge their hearing problems publicly, and this contributes to their social uneasiness and undermines their confidence. "Am I deaf or just dumb?" I've sometimes asked myself, afraid that others may be asking it too.

Psychological "disturbances" are four times greater in the hearing loss population than in the population at large. A 1990 study published in the *Annals of Internal Medicine* found that two-thirds of those with hearing impairments report severe social and emotional handicaps on tests of psychosocial functioning. Patterns of onset of depression seem to correlate with the progression of sensorineural hearing loss. Eventually depression may affect the overall health status of the individual with hearing loss.

The psychological impact can be acute, especially when it's coupled with the cognitive impact of hearing loss. In *The Brain That Changes Itself*, about our increasing understanding of the brain's plasticity, Norman Doidge writes, "When we want to remember something we have heard we must hear it clearly, because a memory can be only as clear as its original signal." The book was published before Frank Lin's epidemiological study of the association between hearing loss and dementia, but it seems to anticipate it.

The depression that comes with losing one of your senses is amplified by the fear of losing your mind. Depression leads to withdrawal, as does the fact that not being able to hear makes you tentative and uncomfortable in social situations. Isolation is a risk factor for dementia. It's a nasty circle.

In 1802, Beethoven wrote eloquently to his brothers Carl and Johann about his deafness. "Oh you men who think or say that I am malevolent, stubborn, or misanthropic, how greatly do you wrong me," he wrote in an anguished plea for understanding. "You do not know the secret cause which makes me seem that way to you . . ." For six years, he wrote, "I have been hopelessly afflicted . . . Though born with a fiery, active temperament, even susceptible to the diversions of society, I was soon compelled to isolate myself, to live life alone."

· · ·

Deafness affects not only the afflicted but family, friends, and coworkers. It puts a strain on relationships with spouses, lovers, children, old friends and new, who are eager to help but find the task unrelentingly difficult. Unacknowledged, hearing loss can cause co-workers to feel that you are shirking your work, are not collegial, or are just bored with the job.

Deafness asks a lot of others. It requires them to speak slowly and to look at you when they speak, to repeat things (sometimes several times), to recognize that you may not remember something because you didn't hear it in the first place. That kind of patience is hard enough for a loving adult partner or a close friend. For a teenage child, for an impatient boss, for a busy doctor, for a stressed Amtrak employee, it may just not be possible. You're dismissed, rebuffed, ignored, treated like a bothersome child. Or the opposite may be true: people talk very slowly, often loudly, condescendingly, demeaningly. You want to scream, "I'm deaf—not dumb!"

One of the hardest situations for me is my book club. It's made up of seven close friends who all know about my hearing loss and try hard to include me. They repeat things I don't hear, and one of them keeps a notebook to write down phrases that I simply can't get. But as one of them said after I'd remarked that a book-club conversation had seemed especially disjointed, "I think that's just what happens during good conversations—you often don't know how you got on a new topic."

That's fine for people who hear, but I need context. Somehow my book club ended up discussing something called Galactic Hamburger. I only know that because the notebook friend wrote the phrase down. To this day, I don't know what it refers to.

• • •

The truly awkward moments occur when I'm with someone I don't want to know about my hearing loss. (This happens less often these days.) I was walking in the park with a friend about three or four months after the implant was activated and just weeks after I'd left my job. We met a longtime acquaintance with his King Charles spaniel. If they say people look like their dogs, they haven't met J., graying and paunchy, and his elegant little dog. I look a lot like my dog—scruffy hair falling in my eyes, a kind of frenetic energy that's a good match for an exuberant puppy.

"How are you liking retirement?" J. asked. His lip curled into a slight sneer. I was deeply unhappy about my "retirement."

"Sorry?" I said.

"How are you liking retirement?" Three times. Finally I turned to my friend.

"Retirement," she said.

"Retirement!" Ah. "I never can quite absorb that word." But even to me it was clear that that was not the only problem.

That panicked moment when you can't hear paralyzes your ability to think. Your mind goes blank. In this case, it was fanned by simmering mutual hostility. J. and I worked in a similar field, and I had landed a job that he was probably more qualified for. That morning in the park, the news of my "retirement" registered on his face as victory. I'd left the *Times*, and not happily. I'd failed. He always knew he could do the job better than me.

Of my job performance, even I have to ask myself, Was I incompetent? Or just deaf? Of the encounter with J., as with many that I found excruciatingly uncomfortable, was I simply being paranoid?

. . .

That spring, around the same time, I went to a book party given by one of my closest friends for a fellow writer. I knew many of the guests by name and e-mail if not by sight, and it should have been fun. In her chatty memoir *Hear Again*, about regaining her hearing after an implant, Arlene Romoff writes how difficult it was to be sociable as she lost her hearing. She describes the hard work of going to a party. "Did I have fun? Not really—I was working too hard."

Even with a hearing aid and implant, I was working too hard. My friend's apartment is enchanting, full of colorful furniture and knickknacks and bare walls painted in vibrant hues. But she has no rugs, no curtains, and there were fifteen or twenty people talking at the same time. The acoustics were overwhelming. I know the tricks to "conversation without hearing," as Romoff puts it. Control the conversation. Ask questions with answers you can anticipate. Position yourself in an area where there's the least amount of noise, lip-read, and then make your brain work. It's exhausting.

I couldn't seem to get a foothold. The sound bounced off the walls and the floors and the ceiling. I couldn't hear people's names, so I didn't know who I was talking to and took wild stabs at follow-up comments and questions. I retreated to my friend's side. She introduced me to the man she was talking to, someone I knew but couldn't place, and of course I missed his name. Twice. After ten minutes I left. I was humiliated, enraged at my condition, and grievously sorry for myself.

. . .

Restaurants are one big minefield for people with hearing loss, from the minute you walk in and ask for your table till the minute you slink out, your head pounding from the effort of trying to keep up with the waiters, your fellow diners, and the choices that seem to come with every course. "What would you like to drink?" a waiter asked Richard Reed, a musician with hearing loss. Reed answered: "Blue cheese dressing."

Why do waiters insist on rattling off the specials when it would be more efficient to hand out a printed daily addition to the regular menu? Maybe it's because so many of them are aspiring actors. I haven't ordered a special in years.

• • •

Sometimes I wish I could wear a sign on my back saying, "I'm deaf."

When someone standing behind me in a crowded store aisle says, "Excuse me," which I don't hear, and then finally, impatiently, gives me a shove.

When I am walking the dog and a jogger comes up behind me. As a puppy, my dog regarded anything running as an invitation to play. Joggers weren't amused. It still startles me if they come too close and I haven't heard them. And he still makes the occasional excited lunge to join them.

When a bicyclist wants to pass and calls out from behind, "On your left!" What?

When I act confused with shopkeepers, according to my daughter, Elizabeth, many things probably run through their minds. As Elizabeth put it when I asked her once: "At first she thought you were another drunk. But then maybe she was just baffled. You're too young to be deaf, too well dressed to be an inarticulate bum, not visibly drunk. Maybe just slow?"

• • •

One of the stories we pursued in my time as theater editor was the abrupt pullout of Jeremy Piven from the David Mamet drama *Speed-the-Plow*, playing a limited run on Broadway. Piven was the marquee name, although his costars Raul Esparza (a much admired stage actor) and Elisabeth Moss (of *Mad Men*) were also audience draws. Piven's performance won praise from *Times* critic Ben Brantley, who wrote of Piven, "He executes [the role] with uncanny grace and intelligence," adding that "He mines a subtler vein, letting you glimpse the genuine, self-questioning weariness beneath Bobby's macho bravado."

The play, which opened on October 24 for a three-month run, sold exceptionally well. Then in mid-December, Piven announced that he was leaving the cast for medical reasons. The producers were apoplectic—Piven was the money tree, the reason the box office was sold out night after night. Broadway was saturated that year with Hollywood imports, intended to draw crowds, and sentiment favored Broadway over the carpetbaggers. Piven's withdrawal played right into this undercurrent of resentment.

Pressured to reveal his medical condition, Piven claimed that he had mercury poisoning from eating too much sushi. It had caused extreme fatigue and his doctor had ordered him to withdraw. Broadway lives by the motto "The show must go on." Sushi? The producers filed a grievance with Actors' Equity against their former star, asking the union to make an independent assessment of the reasons for Piven's departure. The dispute went into arbitration. Piven refused to speak to the press.

And then, on the afternoon in February when the union found in his favor—that he had not violated his contractual obligations—he called Patrick Healy, the *Times* theater reporter, and said he was ready to talk. Piven was known for the role he'd created on HBO's *Entourage*—the arrogant, fast-talking, aggressive agent Ari Gold. His role in *Speed-the-Plow* was similarly arrogant. It was hard to separate the man from his dramatic persona. Patrick met with Piven for an hour or so somewhere outside the office, and then called to say Piven wanted to come in to talk to Healy's editors: Sam Sifton, the culture editor, and me, the theater editor. Another reporter who'd been on the story, Dave Itzkoff, would also be in the meeting.

This was as close to a celebrity scoop as we ordinarily got in Culture, and the office buzzed with anticipation.

My phone rang again. This time it was my mother, uncharacteristically tearful and frightened. My father had seen a surgeon that morning after his lung cancer, in remission for a year, had returned. The news was bad. But even worse than the news was how it was delivered. Brusquely, dismissively, he told my father there was nothing to be done. Sorry. Goodbye. He sent my father home to die. At least that's how my mother described it. The call was stunning, and confusing. Neither my mother nor my father seemed to be saying something that I could absorb, only that the news was very bad.

Minutes later Piven arrived, looking just like Ari Gold, but shorter. He and Sam and Patrick, testosterone pulsing, each for his own reason wanting to be seen by as many people as possible, stopped to talk in the middle of the big open newsroom, an acoustical disaster area. I went over and stood with the others, trying desperately to focus, to catch up on a conversation that was already ahead of me and moving fast, competitive banter bouncing off the glass walls and high ceilings. I felt the panic rising and wondered if I might be sick to my stomach. Whatever hearing I still had was blocked by the muffled roar of anxiety in my head. Moments of extreme stress create intense pressure in my skull, a kind of tinnitus perhaps. Sam turned to me and said something about "Dave." I took a guess and said I'd get him. When I couldn't hear Dave either, I realized I couldn't do it. I asked Dave to tell Sam I'd just gotten upsetting news and had to leave. I went back to my desk and burst into tears.

I could have put the news about my father aside for that moment. But I couldn't put my hearing aside. And my hearing couldn't put my father's prognosis aside. Stress exacerbates hearing loss— and my mother's call caused my hearing to plummet.

• • •

I was so secretive about my hearing loss that even a year after I got my implant, I had almost no contact with other hearing-impaired people. I had read some books, followed some online chats. The books tended to be miracle stories, like Arlene Romoff's *Hear Again*. Romoff is an engaging writer and speaker, clearly an upbeat person, who has done important work in bringing culture, especially theater, to people with hearing loss. But reading her book after I got my implant sent me into despair. She was talking on the telephone after a week! Two years after my implant, I could still barely hear on the phone.

Romoff's progress was so rapid, her awe and wonder at her new life with the implant so unmarred by setback, that her book, intended to be inspirational, made me feel there was something truly wrong with me. I was a failure at the implant. I blamed myself. I didn't try hard enough. I didn't practice enough. I wasn't positive enough. All of this was true. But it is also true that learning to wear a cochlear implant and to hear satisfactorily with it is a long and difficult process. Some never get there, preferring to go back to the easier life of isolation.

It was only when I decided to join the Hearing Loss Association of America that I realized how many people out there were just like me—not only having suffered hearing loss but having a great deal of trouble adjusting to it. I'd hesitated joining. I'm not a joiner. I was reluctant to go to the annual convention, assuming that everyone would know everyone else, would be there with family and friends, and that it was centered around bonding and social activity. There *was* a welcome dinner, an excursion to see *Wicked* at the Kennedy Center. I didn't do those things. But I went to the research symposium, and I went to as many of the individual workshops as I could fit into my schedule. I heard some psychobabble but I also heard a lot of very smart people talking about all aspects of hearing loss, and a lot of smart people in the audience asking questions and making comments.

Many of the workshops were about the psychological impact of hearing loss. I'd been hit hard, but so, I now realized, had many other people. I drank too much, I stopped seeing friends, I stopped going to movies and parties, and eventually, bitterly, left my job. I argued with my children, was impatient with my husband, was short with shopkeepers and others I couldn't understand. Old losses never dealt with commingled with the new. It was a bitter period. By the time I went to the HLAA convention I was beginning to learn to live with my hearing loss, though not yet at peace with it. A year before, mired in depression, I wouldn't have had the initiative to get myself there.

One of the speakers was Jessica Holton, an L.C.S.W. and a clinical addiction specialist. Her talk was titled: "Trying to Escape by Getting Trapped: Using Unhealthy Coping Skills to Grieve Hearing Loss." She was a short woman with a cap of dark hair. Her talk was repetitive and overly simplistic. I almost got up to leave, but I didn't because I realized the reason she was making me uncomfortable was because she was talking about me.

"Grief associated with hearing loss is often misunderstood," she began. "We expect people to grieve quickly. 'It's been three months, you have a nice home, your children are healthy. Get over it.'" This is even more pronounced with hearing loss, because the impact is incomprehensible to most people. Like others, she used the Elisabeth Kubler-Ross model of grieving. "We don't go through the stages one by one. We dance back and forth all the time. The end point is to get to 'This is who I am. This is part of my identity.'"

Getting there is not easy. Holton talked about negative coping skills: drug and alcohol abuse, obsessive behaviors like picking at your skin or pulling on your hair, undereating, overeating, compulsive exercising, jumping from one relationship to another. Anything to assuage the pain. And she talked about how to overcome these and develop positive coping skills.

Sam Trychin, Ph.D., another speaker at the conference, talked about what it is specifically regarding hearing loss that results in such stress. Partly it's the loss of social attachment, partly the daily difficulties of life. "But for most of us, it's the communication problem," he said. "Social attachment is a basic human survival need. The brain grows in response to experience, and the primary stimulus to growth is interaction with others, learning new skills, developing new neurons." Not much happens in developing new neurons, he said, if you're sitting at home watching *Law and Order* reruns.

"How many of you feel pain in the back of the neck or the shoulder area?" he asked. Hands shot up. "Hearing loss and stress affect muscular pain. They also affect the heart rate." He went on to talk about anger, anxiety, depression, embarrassment, frustration, guilt, and shame—what he called "negative highs" (as opposed to "positive highs"). "Negative high produces cortisol from the adrenal gland, which is dumped into the bloodstream." If sustained, it can contribute to heart problems and other major chronic illnesses. A chronic negative high—something that many with hearing loss are familiar with—is "like taking a cortisol bath." It damages your organ system, he said. "If a high level of negative emotion spikes and then goes back down again after twenty minutes or so, it's okay. But if it lasts a week, or if it recurs with frequency even for short periods, this is bad for your health."

In fact, hearing loss and heart disease are statistically related. The Framingham Heart Study found an association between low-frequency hearing loss and a variety of cardiovascular events. David R. Friedland, M.D., Ph.D., professor of otolaryngology and communication sciences at the Medical College of Wisconsin in Milwaukee, hypothesized that low-frequency loss could be an early indication that a patient has cerebrovascular disease or is at risk for cardiovascular disease.

Conventional medical wisdom does not include the ear among the organs associated with cardiovascular risk (the heart, brain, arteries, kidneys, and eyes). But Friedland and his colleagues note that the inner ear is highly vascularized and that damage abnormalities in the stria (nerve fibers) account for low-frequency loss. "Indeed, the inner ear is so sensitive to blood flow that it is possible that any abnormalities in their condition could be noted earlier here than in other parts of the body that are less sensitive."

In his talk, Trychin also noted, "Chronic stress results in confusion, distraction, difficulty making decisions." Even with a carefully annotated date book, I still miss appointments. I forget conversations. I can't remember what I went into the kitchen for. I waffle on decisions. I'm famous (infamous?) in my family for leaving all my options open until the last possible minute.

Finally, Trychin stressed the importance of a strong social network. For me, a new social network is one of the positive outcomes of hearing loss. Deafness—acknowledged, open deafness—has introduced me to people I'd never otherwise have met. A friend in her early sixties said to me recently that she wished she had a way to meet new people. I do.

Accept the fact of hearing loss, Trychin said. Then tell other people about it. There *is* a stigma associated with hearing loss, he said: "incompetent, poor communication skills, damaged, old, infirm, handicapped." The result is "a double whammy. You don't want to admit to it but you constantly fear being found out. Trying to hide it—if you don't wear hearing aids or use assistive listening devices or ask people to speak up—doesn't help. But then, if you do remind them, you have to remind them every thirty seconds. They forget. We're all more interested in what we're saying than in how you are hearing it."

Pretending to be a normal person day after day is exhausting, as the T-shirt—and the calendar and the poster and the coffee mug and the jigsaw puzzle and the bumper sticker—says. Like many clichés, it's true.

VOICES: JAY ALAN ZIMMERMAN

Jay Alan Zimmerman, a composer, turned his hearing loss into the material for *Jay Alan Zimmerman's Incredibly Deaf Musical*, a spirited autobiographical account of his adult-onset hearing loss. On the afternoon I saw his show, there were roars of laughter and recognition, and some tears, among the many people with hearing loss in the audience. (Supertitles projected on the backdrop allowed the people with hearing loss to understand every word.)

Jay and I met for coffee a few months later in our mutual Upper West Side neighborhood. It was mid-afternoon and the café was empty, but he was not able to hear me. He had no hearing aid, and although he's eligible for a cochlear implant he did not have an implant either. I typed my questions for him, and he spoke his answers.

Jay grew up with music. His mother was a piano teacher, as the character called "young Jay" in the musical sings: "Music flew to my cradle/from Mom's piano/As she taught Bach and Chopin/In the room below."

Music became Jay's life as well. He moved to New York and over the next years led what he calls a "diverse hyphenated life." He composed a number of musicals, which won awards and praise from fringe and mainstream groups alike. He was a filmmaker (with a B.F.A. in film from NYU's Tisch School of the Arts). And he appeared in several Off-Off-Broadway productions, as well as doing stand-up comedy. "When music flies the earth spins/And yes, the whole world sings!/It flew from my fingers/From my breath, from my voice," he sings. "All my life I've made it fly/And return back into me/Kept it circling in this endless/Loop of ecstasy."

And then, in 2001 he added another hyphenation: "deaf guy." All this is woven together in *Jay Alan Zimmerman's Incredibly Deaf Musical.* The last two lines of the song quoted above are "But another sound is growing/In a cruel finale!"

In the café that afternoon, Zimmerman described the cruel finale. He and his wife and young son lived in New York in a tiny apartment facing the South Tower of the World Trade Center, their first apartment with a view. They had a "Juliet balcony," he told me—a small balcony big enough for a potted plant—opening onto the living room through a glass door.

On the morning of September 11, he was home alone when he saw papers fluttering around the Twin Towers. He thought it was a ticker tape parade and got out his video camera, and then filmed as first one and later the second tower fell. A whoosh of dust and ash billowed toward him at a tremendous speed. He thought it would break through his glass window, he said, but he was paralyzed, he couldn't move. Instead, it blew open the balcony door, dust and ash and the remains of a building full of people filling the room.

He had always had some trouble hearing—a buzz, a mini mosquito, as he described it—but from that point on, his hearing grew worse. He and his wife and child left the city but the city didn't leave them. He developed numerous respiratory problems that contributed to his hearing loss. His loss was profound above middle C on the piano, but only partially impaired below that. Partly because of this, he was left functionally deaf.

Zimmerman is part of a deaf musician group that gives professional performances—to good reviews—and he continues his theater career. Once a promising young Broadway/Off-Broadway composer, he has learned another way to play and compose music. *Incredibly Deaf Musical* is fast-paced, poignant, and funny. I saw it as part of the New York Musical Theatre Festival, where it was performed six times. At the end, Jay (no longer Jay the character but Jay the composer) leads the audience in a song with supertitles projected behind him. The refrain has the audience, the profoundly deaf with balloons in their hands to enable them to feel the beat, standing and clapping and singing along:

> "You've gotta live with what you've got
> Know what you can change
> And what you cannot
> And if your world falls apart
> Dance in your heart."

SIX

"They Don't Scream, 'I'M WEARING HEARING AIDS!!!' "

This is the way Healthy Hearing, an online hearing aid information source, describes the cosmetic appeal of in-the-ear hearing aids. They're the kind I started with, twenty-three years after they were prescribed. The mean delay between the onset of hearing loss and getting a hearing aid is seven years. Many people never get them at all.

I was fifty-three and acutely aware of my age. Three years before, just after I turned fifty, I had come back to the magazine as deputy editor under Adam Moss, newly promoted himself—and ten years my junior. When the *Times* announced my promotion (and that of Gerry Marzorati, as editorial director), I begged them not to include my age. I wasn't about to blow that discretion and show up with hearing aids. So "invisible" was just right for me.

In the fall of 2002, my hearing dropped to the point where I no longer had a choice. The trigger was again stress. It began with the attack on the World Trade Center and continued, unrelenting, for most of the following year.

I was not near the World Trade Center on 9/11. Like most everyone around the world, I watched the towers fall on television. But the destruction was just a few miles away, with incinerated body parts, scraps of paper, and building debris fluttering down like a grim snowstorm over streets I often walked. In the months following the attack, New York was pervaded by fear and anxiety, about other attacks, anthrax scares, subway threats. There were fighter jets overhead and heavily armored troops on street corners. From my apartment, a few months after, I could look down West End Avenue and see the beams of light that shone into the sky from the World Trade Center site, a tribute that had originated in a cover design commissioned by the *Times Magazine* the week after the attack.

The magazine's offices in the Times Building, then on West Forty-third Street, were on the same floor as the mail room. Every few weeks, men in hazmat suits—white coveralls with hoods and masks—would hurry by, on their way to check a suspicious package. They were protected, but we went on working, vulnerable to whatever menace might be in the air. There were bomb scares. Sometimes the whole building would be evacuated. Sometimes we'd be told to stay on our floor (echoes of the directions given to tenants at the World Trade Center).

It was Elizabeth's first year of high school. She took the subway to East Sixteenth Street every day, transferring at Times Square. I worried constantly about a gas attack on the subway, like the one in Tokyo. I bought her a cell phone and had her call me before she got on the subway and when she got off. The troops in Times Square and throughout the subway system, bristling with guns and body armor, were a daily reminder of the ongoing threat.

Will had just left for college. I was sorry he was away at this moment of national reckoning, but I was relieved he was upstate, away from the bull's-eye. Work was intense as the magazine shifted from features to hard news, focusing on terrorism, war, politics, foreign policy. There was stress at home as well. Things were not going well between Dan and me.

I was too stressed, too distracted, to notice how badly I was hearing. When I went to Dr. Hoffman in the fall of 2002, my hearing test showed serious deterioration in both ears. He recommended hearing aids for both, so finally I followed doctor's orders.

Hearing aids, I quickly learned, can be difficult to fit properly. Therese Deierlein, my audiologist, was unfailingly patient as I tried one brand or fit after another. Each time I tried a new aid, it had to be custom-made for me. Hearing aid companies give you a month to try them out, and getting the whole thing right can take repeated fittings and adjustments. I finally ended up with small red and blue plastic hearing aids. They helped—the right aid actually allowed me to hear better, the left amplified unidentifiable sound but gave me a sense of balance. And they were almost invisible.

. . .

For many people this invisibility allows them to take an important step from denial to acknowledgment. The ads for in-the-ear hearing aids might as well say: "Nobody will ever know you're wearing them! No need to admit the shame of hearing loss!" This stigma, reinforced by the hearing aid companies, is one reason people delay.

Sergei Kochkin of the Better Hearing Institute writes that the delay in getting needed hearing aids can often be lengthy. Some people act quickly, but others wait decades, either until they are no longer able to fool themselves that their hearing is okay or until family or friends finally pressure them into the move. Kochkin notes that the average age of first-time hearing aid users is close to seventy, despite the fact that the majority of people with hearing loss are younger than sixty-five and nearly half of all people with hearing loss are younger than fifty-five.

Frank Lin's 2011 paper finding that 48 million have hearing loss was followed by another that found that only one in seven over fifty uses corrective devices like hearing aids. His study included those with loss in only one ear, which may account in part for the high numbers. Since they could hear with one ear, it was easier to put off getting a hearing aid.

Kochkin worried about the message this study sent. He pointed out that not all people with hearing loss are candidates for hearing aids. By his estimation, when you consider only those who are candidates, the adoption rate is much higher. For those with moderate to severe hearing loss, treatable with hearing aids, the adoption rate is 40 percent. For those in the severe to profound category, the rate of adoption is 60 to 65 percent. Kochkin was concerned that Lin's conclusions could backfire, resulting in even less rather than more hearing aid use. "I think the Hopkins data does a great disservice from a PR perspective by reporting such low [misleading] adoption rates . . . Who wants to be an outlier and adopt hearing aids with those low figures?"

Even though only one in seven over fifty who could benefit from a hearing aid uses one, the preponderance of users are indeed elderly (thus reinforcing the stigma of age). Frank Lin's study found that only 4.5 percent of those aged fifty to fifty-nine who need hearing aids use them, whereas 22.1 percent over eighty do. I asked Lin if this was the result of a reluctance to wear hearing aids on the part of younger people (the aging stigma) or whether he had accounted for the degree of hearing loss in making the comparisons. Both are partly true. ("Great question," he wrote in an e-mail. I love being complimented for my astuteness.) "Yes indeed, fifty-year-olds have less severe hearing loss than eighty-plus [people], which definitely accounts to some extent for the lower rate of hearing aid use. But if you look at the table, rates of hearing aid use for each age group, *after stratifying by hearing loss severity levels*, shows that fifty-year-olds are a lot less likely to use hearing aids compared to the oldest adults."

The relatively low rate of use in the U.K., where hearing aids are free, supports the notion that stigma plays a role. Although Sergei Kochkin initially disagreed with this assessment, writing in an e-mail that the adoption rate has much more to do with degree of hearing loss than with the stigma of age, a 2007 MarkeTrak study disputes that finding: "Table 2 shows that non-adopter mean average ages are between 8 and 15 years lower than those of typical non-users. What can account for the difference in age between the typical hearing aid user and the non-adopter? It is our theory that age stigma accounts for a significant amount of the factors explaining hearing aid adoption."

• • •

It's not just vanity. In the United States hearing aids are expensive. Fitted in-the-ear hearing aids, the kind that work best for people with mild to moderate loss, are very expensive. This is the kind I started with. As my hearing worsened, I moved up to behind-the-ear with a fitted in-the-ear component. Mild to moderate impairment is a degree of loss people may be able to live with. For this group, hearing aids are often put in the category of discretionary spending, a quality-of-life purchase.

Insurance companies also consider hearing aids discretionary quality-of-life purchases, no matter how severe your hearing loss is. Most private insurers classify them as medical devices and either refuse to cover them or reimburse at a rate that is a fraction of the cost. Since uncorrected hearing is associated with job loss and psychological problems, this may not be a cost-effective strategy.

The cost of a good hearing aid ranges from $2000 to $6000. Some accuse audiologists and manufacturers of unconscionable markups. The truth is—of course—more complex, but the bottom line is that they cost an enormous amount of money. Recently Congress proposed a tax on hearing aids as part of the health care reform bill. In the end, hearing aids (as well as eyeglasses and contact lenses) were declared exempt.

Despite the cost, a hearing aid is easy to misplace. You take it off in a noisy place or because your ear is tired or the battery has failed. Ideally, you're carrying the case it goes in. I never seem to have it. I tuck the hearing aid into my bra. This has a couple of unfortunate consequences: The first is that it sometimes creates a bump under my shirt that looks like an oddly placed nipple. The second is that I often throw bra and hearing aid into the laundry basket.

Stories of people eating their hearing aids may be apocryphal. One man of my acquaintance, his wife says, put his on the edge of his plate in a noisy restaurant and later popped it into his mouth, thinking it was a crust of bread (we don't know if he actually swallowed it). A woman in Idaho gained Internet fame when she mistook hers for a Milk Dud. Stories of dogs eating hearing aids are common. I've lost a cell phone, countless watchbands, and a pair of glasses to my dog. Not the hearing aid—yet. (In 2012, the dog did eat my implant earpiece. Advanced Bionics replaced it under the onetime irreparable damage or loss policy.)

Along with cost, discomfort, stigma, and how easy hearing aids are to misplace is the fact that often they don't work very well. We've made great progress since the days when hearing aids screeched and whistled, but they are still far from foolproof in detecting speech. They're also difficult for clumsy or aging fingers to manipulate. The battery is a minuscule disk that the user fits into a small hinged door. My fingers aren't clumsy or aging, but I often drop the battery when I'm trying to insert it. It goes bouncing off under a piece of furniture and I never see it again.

Women are more likely to have hearing aids and cochlear implants than men. There are probably many reasons for this, among them that hearing aids are not as visible under long hair, but also women are famously better at taking care of themselves than men.

• • •

Part of being an audiologist is talking to the patient as you try out the hearing aids, calibrating them in response to what the patient is hearing. Therese, my audiologist, talks like a tape recorder set on "fast." Turn the "on" switch and the words tumble out, punctuated here and there by "Is this too loud?" and "How does my voice sound?" I say "fine," or "too loud," and she resumes where she left off. Over the years I learned all about her nephews' successful garage band, her favorite restaurants, the plays she's seen. She always remembers, even when months go by between visits, to ask me about my husband, my kids, my dog, my work.

Therese is preternaturally pale, thin, with glasses halfway down her nose and wiry gray-blond hair that she fruitlessly tries to control with a barrette. It seems as if all her energy, every bit of nutrition she gets (though it's hard to see when she has time to eat, since she's in the office from eight till eight many days), turns into multi-tasking—speed-dialing a hearing aid company on speakerphone to ask a question, meanwhile programming my hearing aid on her computer, asking me about what movies I've seen, reaching behind her to get a device she wants to show me. When she leaves a message on my phone, she talks so fast that the only way I know it's Therese is by looking at the caller ID.

For those first hearing aids, she fitted me with two small Widex digital devices. "Fitting" is nothing like Bergdorf's custom-altering a dress for you, though it's a lot more expensive. The audiologist mixes a paste from green-and-white squishy silicone and injects it into your ear with a big syringe. It sits there for five minutes or so, cold and uncomfortable, and then, when it's hardened, she pulls it out by a string. The mold and your hearing specifications are sent off to the manufacturer, and a week or so later your hearing aid comes back. Sometimes it fits. Sometimes you have to do the whole squishy fitting all over again.

Whenever I first put on a new hearing aid, or a newly calibrated one, it sounds unbearably loud and my own voice sounds even louder. Therese manipulates some dials on her computer—"How does this sound?" "Is my voice too loud?" "How's your dog?" "How are the higher-pitched sounds?" "Have you seen . . . ?" "Last Saturday I went to . . ." "Is this better?" Finally we settle on an acceptable level and I leave the office to try it out in the real world for a couple of weeks. Stepping out onto the street is an assault. It's so noisy! But even as I walk the seven blocks south to the subway, my ear—or my brain—begins to adjust and the noise subsides. Within an hour or so I am hearing fairly normally. I quickly learned that whenever my hearing aid is reprogrammed, I have to have Therese set it a little too loud, because I will adjust in a few hours and then it will be too soft.

The ruby-red Widex in the right ear did all the work. The sapphire in the left served only to give me a sense of sound binaurally and help me orient myself. I went back to Therese every two weeks for the first few months while she fiddled with the programming. After that, I saw her for regular programming visits once every three months, and sometimes for panicked emergencies. One time I was sure I had lost the tiny plastic "wax guard" (intended to protect the inner electronics from earwax) inside my ear. In fact, I thought I might have lost several of them. I imagined little white plastic pinheads rolling around inside my ear.

Other times I just felt that something was wrong, and she'd fix it. I never paid Therese for the many visits I made to her over the years. The cost was folded into the cost of the hearing aid. I had to upgrade to new aids several times, but she couldn't have been making money on me—I was way too labor-intensive.

● ● ●

These days, many people are able to wear "open-fit" hearing aids, sleek metallic crescents that sit snugly behind the ears, with colors that match almost any hair color, connected by a thin plastic tube to a very small in-the-ear component. They are much easier to fit because the in-the-ear component floats rather than molds itself to the ear opening. The open-fit style works well for mild to moderate hearing loss, requires a less extensive fitting process, and provides more natural sound quality since the ear is not entirely blocked.

My hearing loss was too severe for the open-fit design. I have the same sleek behind-the-ear crescent and invisible plastic tubing, but the in-the-ear component is the size of a fat thumb. I've had my current hearing aid for three years as I'm writing this and, alas, I've maxed out on this one too. I'm about to upgrade once again.

Each upgrade is a grueling process. I often go through four or five hearing aids before I find one I'm comfortable with. In each case, Therese makes a mold with the squishy green stuff, the manufacturer creates a hearing aid, I wear it for a few weeks. And I send it back.

Despite careful fitting and repeated adjustments, the hearing aids would become uncomfortable over the course of a long day, and they inevitably amplified unwanted noise. My ears would get tired wearing them—a condition known as hearing aid fatigue— and I'd take them off. If I was at work, I'd shove them under a pile of papers or drop them in my pocket—furtively, anything to keep people from noticing. If I'd forgotten to flick open the battery door when I took one off, it would whistle. (This is presumably to remind the user that the battery is still on. I can't hear it myself, but it serves to drive dogs and hearing humans crazy.) Someone would comment, "What's that noise?" I knew what noise it was and would discreetly flip open the battery door with my fingernail.

In noisy places, like a restaurant, I heard better without the hearing aids—at least for a while. Eventually I couldn't hear in a restaurant with or without them. I'd read lips and hope for the best.

• • •

Even in quiet conditions—even with my hearing aids—there were people whose voices were pitched at a level that I simply lacked the ability to hear. My magazine colleague Alex Star would come into my office, and though the acoustics were optimal, I still couldn't hear him. I was deep in the faking-it stage of loss—past denial but not yet ready to be completely open about it. Recently I asked Alex if he had noticed.

He said I had told him about the loss. "I did notice that you often held back at meetings, and didn't necessarily engage in conversational back-and-forth after you'd given your own assessment of a piece," he wrote in an e-mail.

"I recognized a certain reticence in your approach to the job. I could see from your reading of our knottier science stories that your analytic gifts were considerable, and yet I sensed a reluctance to use them fully in face-to-face interactions. I attributed this reticence to temperament, or to a discomfort with the management of the magazine, or to that all too common phenomenon: a waning of interest in the workaday routines of journalism after years in the trenches."

I read this e-mail with a combination of enlightenment and humiliation. Alex had put his finger on an aspect of hearing loss that is far more destructive than simply not hearing or mishearing. After a while, as your hearing loss worsens and you've made one blunder after another, you become wary, reluctant to take chances in conversation. Your confidence is undermined. You may express a bold and even controversial idea if you're the original speaker, but once the conversation turns into a discussion, with questions, challenges, new ideas and thoughts, you shrink back, hoping no one will notice.

It got to the point that I was conscious of the loss every time someone spoke to me and I couldn't follow what was said, every time I flinched at the too-loud clatter of dishes or the grinding of a garbage truck, every time I couldn't hear dialogue at the theater or a movie, every time the phone rang and I struggled to identify the caller, every time someone tried to tell me something confidentially, lowering his or her voice so as not to be overheard. It was a loss that could never be tucked away, stuffed in a drawer, forcibly pushed into the background.

Even in a crisis, my hearing thrust its way forward. After my husband had cancer surgery, my focus was on *hearing* the surgeon, rather than listening to what he said. When the EMS came in response to a crisis involving my mother, the overwhelming issue was *hearing* their words, not what the words meant. A transportation glitch—a stalled subway, a grounded plane—was not about being delayed or trapped or claustrophobic. It was about the fact that I couldn't hear what anyone was saying—not only announcements but also even speculation from fellow passengers. I was often reduced to tears of frustration, and sometimes I panicked, unable to ask for help—because I couldn't hear the answer—or to help myself.

In September 2011, a British couple was kidnapped from their luxury safari camp in Kenya. The man was killed, but the woman was taken hostage. She was described as being "severely hearing impaired." I dwelt on the nightmare of being blindfolded and not able to hear, the hearing aid batteries gone dead. Hostages often describe the sounds they heard as a way of identifying their captors or the place they were taken. But also as a way of assuring themselves that they were still alive.

The only time I ever forgot about my hearing was when I was asleep, at which point it could be something of an advantage. I could theoretically sleep through anything. But I didn't. Anxiety and depression kept me awake for what seemed like ten years.

• • •

To casual acquaintances and even to some of my closest friends, I seemed to be doing well, and I was, relatively speaking. But, harking back to the Seattle psychoanalyst Jacqui Metzger's comment about the fragility of "acceptance" of one's hearing loss, there were, and continue to be, difficult moments. Getting a new hearing aid is one of them. For all the times I've been fitted with a new aid, I continue to find the process as surprisingly draining as it was the first time around.

Ten years after getting those first hearing aids, I was still working with Therese. The visits were no less intense, and sometimes dispiriting. In the fall of 2011, I went to Therese because I had come to realize that some of the devices she'd offered me over the years (that I'd pushed away as just too much stuff to deal with) actually might improve my hearing. I wanted an FM system, which allows a speaker's voice to be transmitted directly to my hearing aid and implant. Jacqui Metzger had one, and that was how she was able to treat psychoanalytic patients she couldn't see.

I was also interested in being able to use the new technology called looping. A hearing loop system consists of a thin strand of copper wire installed on the floor around the periphery of a room or an auditorium or theater or church. It can be more creatively installed by weaving it around rows of seats, which produces better results, especially in a theater. It transmits the audio information (speech, music, etc.) picked up by a microphone, or wired into the amplifier from a music player, via an electromagnetic signal. People with telecoils pick up the sound directly in their hearing aid or implant. Those without telecoils can utilize hearing loop technology by wearing special headphones.

Hearing loop technology is common in Western Europe and in the Midwest, but rare in New York and other East Coast cities. An article by John Tierney, "A Hearing Aid That Cuts Out All the Clatter," which appeared in the *Times* in October 2011, was the first many on the East Coast had heard of looping. The Kennedy Center in Washington, D.C., has occasionally installed a loop system temporarily, as other venues also do, but very few have permanent looping. Installing a loop system, according to the *Times* article, typically costs $10 to $25 a seat.

Unlike the infrared headsets offered at New York theaters and other venues, hearing loops are both invisible and effective. Infrared headsets, as the hearing aid ads say, scream "I'm hard of hearing!" They also don't work for those with severe hearing loss. I tried the infrared device at a performance of *August: Osage County*, a dialogue-heavy play, and replaced the headset with my hearing aid after the first act.

The hearing aid I was using in the fall of 2011 did not have the telecoil needed for looping. But by then I wasn't hearing well out of it anyway, so Therese ordered me a Widex with a telecoil.

When it came, it was completely the wrong fit. A glitch at the manufacturer. She sent it back.

A week later, I returned with high hopes for the new Widex. Better speech clarity was my primary concern. I also hoped for better phone clarity. When I tried it out, and after she'd adjusted the programming, I felt like I was hearing no better than I had with the old aid. Then I tried making a phone call using the telecoil. The minute she switched on the telecoil program the hearing aid started buzzing, a response to the fluorescent light fixture above us. The phone call was clear enough through the buzzing, but so is

listening with the Bluetooth device (called an iCom) that I use with
my Phonak hearing aid. It didn't seem like much of an improvement, especially not one I wanted to pay thousands of dollars for.

Therese decided the Widex had the wrong "algorithm" and ordered an upgraded Phonak. She also said that she could get me an
FM system that would work with my iCom Bluetooth transmitter,
by attaching a small receiver to the bottom. I was impatient and
tired, and said I couldn't see any reason to order the new hearing
aid until I tried out the old one with the FM. But the iCom itself
wasn't working properly and had to go back to the manufacturer, so
I had to wait till it was fixed to try the FM. The handheld remote
I use to program the hearing aid had also gone dead. It too went
back to the manufacturer. So, essentially, did my hearing.

I canceled appointments and postponed a visit to my mother in
South Carolina. The whole experience—the hearing aid snafus and
the fact that they never would be like normal hearing; the implant
I had gotten in 2009, which I was not doing well with—combined
to defeat me, at least for the moment. Here I am, I thought, thirty-
four years after losing my hearing, ten years after getting hearing
aids, and still struggling. What do others like Arlene Romoff and
Michael Chorost, who have written about their success with cochlear implants, have that I don't? More determination, more grit,
more focus on making it work? Or maybe it's just that their cases
are simpler: no hearing aid/implant combo to muddy the auditory
waters. Even if I don't use my hearing aid, the little I do hear in my
right ear overrides the implant in my left and makes it less effective
than it should be.

The next week I geared myself up to try again, and (probably
foolishly) began to hope that maybe this time—with a new hearing
aid and the SmartLink FM system—I'd be able to hear well enough
to pay attention to what was being said instead of simply whether
I was hearing it.

Because of further snafus, neither the new hearing aid nor the
FM system worked. In fact, nothing worked with anything else.

A problem of connectivity and technology. Back to the manufacturer. By now it was the holidays, and everything was put on hold
for another few weeks.

I invited fifteen people to Christmas dinner. By Christmas, the
number had expanded to twenty-four. (Do you mind if I bring
my mother? Could I bring my roommate who's alone in the city?
My sister and her husband? My boyfriend?) I enjoyed Christmas on
non-auditory levels: seeing the multiple generations around my table, using my mother's beautiful silver and china that she had passed
on to me when she moved to a smaller place, feeling the goodwill
and cheer, eating good food and drinking good wine. There were
toasts and hugs, and a long comfortable lingering end to the evening around the remains of dinner. Hearing played a minor role, but
sight, taste, smell, touch all enjoyed themselves immensely.

• • •

An FM system is like "a miniature personal FM radio station," as
Brad Ingrao, a well-known audiologist who is often invited to speak
at hearing loss conferences, described it. The speaker holds the transmitter, or wears it on a loop around his neck, and talks normally. The
transmitter can also be put on the podium at a lecture, or in the
middle of the table at a dinner (if it's quiet enough and only one person speaks at a time). The listener wears a receiver, which communicates the sound to the telecoil in the hearing aid or implant. Ideally,
you hear the speaker's voice clearly through hearing aid or implant
or both, with background noise screened out.

It took me quite a while to get all my FM equipment configured,
something made especially difficult by my having both a hearing
aid and a cochlear implant. It turned out the cochlear implant
would not work with the Bluetooth, only with a transmitter called a
MyLink. Eventually, a month or two later, I ended up with a new
hearing aid with a telecoil, so my FM receiver now feeds the signal
from the transmitter/microphone combo to both the hearing aid
and the cochlear implant via the single receiver. The transmitter also

allows me (theoretically—I haven't gotten it to work yet, so I still use the iCom) to pair Bluetooth devices like my cell phone and MP3 player, and I can plug it into the TV so that for the first time in years I can hear without captions.

My daily equipment now includes hearing aid, implant, Smart-Link (the FM system), and MyLink. The MyLink connects the SmartLink wirelessly to hearing aid and implant. They all need to be charged at least once a day. I travel with a power strip.

Here's the irony, though. Once I got all this set up, I went to a lecture for the first time in many years. E. O. Wilson was being interviewed at the New York Public Library and I was very excited about hearing him talk. I did hear him talk—I heard almost every word. But I discovered that I have lost the ability to listen. After years of absorbing oral information visually—through subtitles— I can no longer absorb it without the visual crutch. It's the same old cognitive deficit—my brain is working too hard on hearing the words to listen to what's being said.

VOICES: RICHARD EINHORN

"I was one of maybe fifteen or twenty people in the United States who had one of those 'golden ears,'" Richard Einhorn told me. "I could go into a concert hall and clap my hands and know whether or not it was appropriate to record classical music."

Richard Einhorn is a former classical music record producer and an accomplished composer. His *Voices of Light*, inspired by the classic silent film *The Passion of Joan of Arc*, has been performed by many major symphony orchestras. In the early nineties he developed otosclerosis in both ears. The three small bones that carry vibrations to the inner ear fused together and no longer vibrated properly. A surgeon replaced the bones in his right ear with a plastic prosthesis.

He heard well in that ear for some time. But in June 2010, without any warning or known cause, he lost all functional hearing in his right ear. That ear went, as he says, dead. He hears nothing but "unbelievably distorted" noise, a condition known as recruitment. He wears an earplug in that ear. In his left ear, he hears with a hearing aid. But in noisy situations he takes his hearing aid out, places a $500 Shure earbud into his ear, and plugs the earbud into an iPhone running an app called soundAMP R.

Richard Einhorn continues to compose. Like most composers, he essentially hears the music in his head. He can't hear stereo (because of the right-ear loss) but, he says, "I can imagine stereo very easily. So I'm fine."

Einhorn has found his own way around the complications and confusions of assistive technology. He sympathized with my trouble trying to coordinate implant and hearing aid and assistive devices meant for one or the other. "Why is it all so complicated?" he said. "Where is the Steve Jobs of hearing loss?"

SEVEN

And Then You Have to Pay for It

For most people the primary obstacle to buying hearing aids—not to mention hearing-assistive technology like the iCom or Zoom-Link—is cost. There's no question that they're expensive, and in fact out of reach for many people. Many people need two (partly because so much hearing loss is noise induced, and tends to be binaural).

It's easy to understand the distrust people feel about hearing aid companies when you can buy a sophisticated smartphone for $500 or a MacBook Pro for $1300; a digital camera, an iPod that holds hundreds of thousands of songs and movies, a huge flat-screen TV—each for a fraction of the price of a single hearing aid.

An angry letter from someone named Brenda D. Shanley in response to an article on hearing aids on Hearing Loss Web (an invaluable compendium of news about technology, policy, advances, and everything to do with hearing aids and cochlear implants) addressed the issue of price gouging. Whereas the "normal, 'average' pricing wholesale to retail in most industries other than hearing aids is double the cost," she claimed, in the hearing aid industry "the markup is TEN TIMES the cost. What cost $100 will be sold retail for $1000."

An audiologist responded to Shanley, calling these allegations "absolutely untrue" and "completely absurd." "Jan," as she identified herself, is not only a dispenser of hearing aids, but a consumer, for her daughter. She went on to say that her markup often isn't enough to cover costs. These include not just the wholesale price of the hearing aid but "the time I spend with customers on training, setting, resetting, remaking, troubleshooting, making impressions, new impressions, sending in for repairs, selling batteries etc. etc." She added that most of the hearing aids she orders cost at least $1000 wholesale, and pointed out that if she were selling them at a ten times markup, they'd cost $10,000.

I was shocked by the cost of hearing aids, and outraged that they were not covered by my health insurance. But I never felt cheated. I spend an average of one hour per visit to the audiologist for fitting, calibrating, cleaning, counseling, discussing hearing-assistive technology like Bluetooths and FM systems (which themselves require maintenance and training), and occasionally having a hearing test. The cost of these follow-up visits is included in the original cost of the hearing aid, just as the costs of maintenance or repair or training with the Bluetooth or FM system are rolled into the original cost of those devices.

As of January 2012, all newly certified audiologists are required to have a Ph.D. (Certification also requires a minimum of 1820 hours of supervised clinical work.) Clearly, audiologists don't go into the profession for the money. The median annual income for an audiologist in 2008, according to the Bureau of Labor Statistics, was $62,030. For optometrists it was $96,320, for physical therapists $72,900. Those are median income figures—an audiologist in private practice in an urban area may well earn over $100,000, but the same increased income is true for optometrists and physical therapists.

Despite that $2000-to-$6000 figure, the cost of hearing aids has actually decreased relatively over time when compared to the rate of inflation, according to an article in Healthy Hearing in April 2010. The article noted the factors that contribute to the high cost: research and development, manufacturing costs, customization of the hearing aid to fit the needs of the consumer, and time spent with the professional (the audiologist). "Averaged over the lifetime of the instruments (three to five years or more), the cost per day of a pair of hearing aids is about three dollars."

John Niparko, then director of the Division of Otology, Audiology, Neurotology and Skull Base Surgery at Johns Hopkins (he is now at USC), addressed the issue of research and development costs in an interview at Hopkins in the spring of 2011. "We're always ten to fifteen years behind cellular and laptop technology because our markets are literally 1 percent of those markets," he said. "So when a cell phone maker wants to design a new phone, they will order five million transistors or chips to run it—chips are really the name of the game now. We'll order ten thousand; I mean, there's just no comparison. It's just a completely different scale." Even with demographics predicting a much greater demand for hearing aids, there will still be no competition. The numbers will go up, he said, "but not like they will for cell phone use, where more than half the population owns a cell phone."

And not just any cell phone. A 2012 Pew Research survey found 46 percent of Americans owned a smartphone, and the numbers are growing rapidly. According to statistics compiled by Gartner research that same year, 65 percent of the U.S. population is expected to own a smartphone or smart tablet by 2015. *The Guardian* reported in the fall of 2011 that half of the U.K. population owned a smartphone (with Google's Android claiming half the market, followed by the BlackBerry and the iPhone).

Adding insult to financial injury is the lack of insurance coverage for hearing aids. When insurance does pay, it's generally $500 or less. Medicare does not reimburse for hearing aids, except under certain circumstances. Medicaid reimbursement varies from state to state. Hearing tests for infants are mandatory, but insurance does not always cover hearing aids for children—this seems not only counterproductive but ridiculous. The Affordable Care Act does not cover hearing aids.

The IDEA (Individuals with Disabilities Education Act) ensures equal education for children with hearing impairment or other disabilities. But unless children are fitted with hearing aids (or cochlear implants) when they are prelingual, they may have severe developmental speech difficulties (unless they use ASL). Children also outgrow their hearing aids rapidly, often after just a few months. Some states maintain hearing aid loaner banks for children.

Flexible spending accounts, sometimes offered as part of an employer-sponsored insurance plan, allow employees to take up to $5000 tax free per family out of the insured employee's gross salary to pay for medical expenses, which can include hearing aids. (In January 2013, the amount will be reduced to $2500.) But this is your own money you're spending—all you're saving is the tax you would have paid on that portion of your income. Moreover, only 20 percent of U.S. employees contributed to a flexible spending account in 2010, and most contributed significantly less than the upcoming $2500 maximum. The savings ranged from $250 to $640 a year in taxes.

A hearing aid tax credit reintroduced in the House in April 2011 would allow an income tax deduction of $500 per hearing aid for seniors over fifty-five and for dependents as defined by the IRS, with one deduction allowed every five years. H.R. 1479 looks unlikely to pass Congress this session, as similar bills have failed in earlier years. The comments on WashingtonWatch.com on this issue are surprisingly offensive.

The response to a woman who commented in favor of the bill, who had two children with hearing aids at a total cost well over $10,000, was: "You think that qualifies you for a tax break? WHY? If that's true I should have a tax break for my hangnails too. VOTE NO!"

Another writer, named Priscilla, wrote: "I am a seventy-two-year-old and a cancer survivor. My hearing got dramatically worse after chemo. Hearing aids to improve this loss cost approximately 5000 dollars. The tax credit would help make this more affordable.

Please vote yes on the tax credit." Another commentator character-ized comments like hers as "just more welfare whine. VOTE NO!"

The provision for a $500 reimbursement remains in limbo, but a bill to make the cost of hearing aids a legitimate medical expense and therefore tax deductible passed.

. . .

The consumer does have some options, other than putting off the purchase as long as possible. Buying hearing aids online has be-come popular, accounting for an increasingly large percentage of the market. Sellers range from reputable to irresponsible; buyer beware. Direct-mail sales have also increased. Audiologists bemoan the trend (and not just because it takes business away from them), and the FDA warns that it may be harmful. Online retailers include vendors like eBay and Amazon.com—which call some of their prod-ucts "hearing aids," though most, more accurately, are referred to as "personal sound amplifiers."

Internet sites like HearingPlanet.com and americahears.com require the buyer to have a professional hearing test at either an audiologist or an ENT, in compliance with FDA regulations. Hear ingPlanet.com refers customers to its own local clinics. America hears.com says, "We strongly recommend that you see an Ear, Nose and Throat physician for a medical examination and complete hearing evaluation to determine your need for a hearing instru-ment." (Consumers can also waive their rights and skip the test, though both sites discourage that.)

Among the reasons not to buy online, from a company that does not offer professional services, are, first, that the risk of an in-appropriate fit is high. In addition, the manufacturers' proprietary formulas for calculating amplification requirements, commonly known as "first fit" formulas, are often not right for the user. Getting the correct amplification may require returning hearing aids to the company for adjustments, perhaps several times.

Suzanne H. Kimball of Illinois State University conducted

some real-world evaluations of online hearing aid purchases. First she tested online hearing tests. Eighty-one subjects in three age groups took both an online hearing test and a hearing test in a hearing test suite. Results showed "statistically significant differences between the results of the online and professional testing conditions," she wrote in a report in *Hearing Journal*. The older participants, not surprisingly, had a harder time negotiating the online test. Individual differences between the two test conditions ranged from 10 to 40 decibels, with some as great as 85 decibels.

As Kimball points out, consumers fitted with hearing aids after an online test might not only get an inappropriate fit but actually place themselves at risk for further hearing damage if the levels are set too high. Many online hearing tests have a quirk that can skew results: as soon as the subject presses yes (meaning the tone has been heard), the computer immediately moves on to a lower-intensity signal, thus allowing the subject to anticipate the signal simply by timing, whether consciously or not. In a hearing booth, the audiologist randomizes the time between signals.

The following year, Kimball, this time with Susan Yopchick, compared fittings online with fittings done in an audiologist's office. There were only two subjects in this test. "The hearing aids bought online were poorly fitted for both patients," the authors wrote. The first subject was a seventy-one-year-old woman who had been diagnosed with sudden sensorineural hearing loss ten years earlier. "She brought to our clinic a bag full of the ear molds that have been made for her over the years," saying that she used most of them, hearing better with one ear mold one day and another on another day. She was a tough case. After trying five pairs of clinically fitted ear molds, she returned to her original hearing aids. The online ear molds (based on an ear mold her husband had taken) were comfortable, but she couldn't hear very well with them and was tired of racking up $30 shipping and insurance fees, and eventually she returned them to the company.

The second subject was a fifty-seven-year-old man who had never worn a hearing aid. The online test indicated a mild hearing loss in one ear and moderate in the other (the opposite of what was established in the clinic). He was offered a choice of approximately sixty hearing aids and picked one, marketed as 100 percent digital and costing $499.50. After wearing it for a few hours a day during the trial period, he eventually decided it was too loud and returned the aid. The clinic recommended binaural open-fit BTE hearing aids. He reportedly wears them inconsistently but is satisfied with them.

Much of the population of people with hearing loss is over sixty-five, and 40 percent of people with hearing loss of all ages have mild to moderate hearing loss. The majority of purchasers are older and likely to be on a fixed income, with perhaps little to spare for a $3000 hearing aid. Some decide they'll just hear poorly, accepting it as a part of aging. Others go to cheaper outlets. The debate over direct-mail or direct-to-seller hearing aids or hearing aids bought online has continued for almost a decade.

When I first heard about hearing aids online, I was skeptical. I spend hours and hours with my audiologist, getting just the right fit and calibrations. But I have severe to profound hearing loss and my hearing aid needs are not those of most hearing aid consumers. I'm a working professional and need to be able to communicate under many different circumstances. Of necessity I wear a fitted, in-the-ear hearing aid, with a behind-the-ear component. This means that the in-the-ear part must fit perfectly or else it will be uncomfortable or ineffective.

But for those with less severe hearing loss, a behind-the-ear hearing aid, with a small device in the ear that does not need an ear-mold fitting, works quite well and is nearly invisible. These can be bought online, as can in-the-ear devices. With in-the-ear devices, the consumer is sent the material to make the mold and does it at home.

PreciseHearing.com, which can be linked to from Amazon.com,

offers the Siemens Pure 301 Behind-the-Ear Hearing aid for $1149 (regular price $1349). Amazon itself no longer seems to sell hearing aids, though they did until quite recently. Hearing Revolution, an online retailer, sells the similar Siemens Pure 701 for $1995. Hearing Revolution also features articles about hearing aids, including one titled "Buyers Beware: Ordering Hearing Aids Off the Internet," posted on March 24, 2011, by Kristin Slifer, Au.D. These are behind-the-ear hearing aids, so there is no fitting required, as there would be with in-the-ear hearing aids. The hearing aid is programmed at Siemens, based on an audiogram done by a qualified audiologist.

At the other end of the spectrum are a variety of cheap rechargeable hearing aids, meaning no fumbling with minuscule batteries. Charles D. Hornbrook ("Buckeye") of Suwannee, Florida, self-described as a "big guy, 6 ft, 225 lbs, wear size 12E boots and XXL gloves," was, to put it mildly, unhappy with the product he bought, the Infini Ear ITE, which sold for $39.95. He ordered the larger size. "They almost fit in my ear, but are so large that just walking across the room causes them to fall out because they cannot be inserted far enough and they are 'outboard heavy.'" He added, among a total of nine complaints: "Nearly Invisible? Mine look like someone stuck a large 1″ × 5/8″ mushroom in my ear."

The FDA defines a hearing aid as "any wearable [sound-amplifying] instrument or device designed for, offered for the purpose of, or represented as aiding persons with or compensating for, impaired hearing." In order to buy a product labeled a hearing aid, "a prospective hearing aid user must provide to the hearing aid dispenser a written statement from a licensed physician that the prospective user has been medically evaluated and is a candidate for a hearing aid. This evaluation must occur within 6 months prior to the date of purchase of the hearing aid. If 18 years of age or older, the prospective user may waive this requirement for medical evaluation provided that the prospective user signs a waiver statement under the conditions outlined in this regulation. Children (age less than 18 years) are not eligible for a waiver."

Many people with mild hearing loss instead buy "personal sound amplification products," or PSAPs. These devices do not require a physician's statement, since, as the FDA says, "PSAPs are intended to amplify environmental sound for non-hearing-impaired consumers. They are not intended to compensate for hearing impairment." They are also not classified as medical devices under the Food, Drug, and Cosmetic Act, and thus are not eligible for tax exemptions. Eric Mann, deputy director of the FDA's Division of Ophthalmic, Neurological and Ear, Nose and Throat Devices, warns that choosing a PSAP for hearing loss without consulting a physician "can cause a delay in diagnosis of a potentially treatable condition."

The Better Hearing Institute's database on the hearing loss population, MarkeTrak VIII (2008–2009), found that 3.28 percent of hearing aid owners had bought their hearing aids by direct mail. The survey also found that these subjects wore their hearing aids a median of three hours a day (compared to custom-hearing-aid wearers, who wore them ten hours per day). Direct-mail purchasers and those who bought PSAPs were more than twice as likely as custom-hearing-aid users to have unilateral loss and a greater tendency to describe their hearing loss as mild. Income level among the PSAP users averaged $10,000 less than that of custom users. Only 17.8 percent of these users said they would have purchased custom hearing aids if PSAPs were not available.

These devices are probably fine for people with mild hearing loss (as long as they've made sure there is no underlying disease) but the MarkeTrak VIII survey also found that among those using PSAPs, 10 percent were in the highest decile for hearing loss. If your hearing loss is in the fifth decile or higher (the top 60 percent of people with hearing loss), you probably need custom-fitted and calibrated hearing aids. Almost 80 percent of direct-mail buyers and 72 percent of PSAP owners are candidates for custom hearing aids because of the severity of their loss.

• • •

Direct-to-consumer retailers (like Lloyds, which has been in operation for over forty-five years), Americahears.com and HearSource .com offer hearing aids, usually with the programming done at home by the consumer using software provided by the retailer. Songbird, also a direct-to-consumer outlet, offered a disposable hearing aid, "perfect for anyone with mild to moderate hearing loss, especially those who don't need hearing help all the time." Songbird hearing aids ranged in price from $99 to $299.90. The company has gone out of business.

The third and most popular alternative to an independent audiology clinic is retail outlets, often the big box stores. Amplifon USA is the largest hearing aid retailer in the country and is the parent company of both the Amplifon Hearing Centers, which are located in Wal-Mart Supercenters, and of Miracle-Ear, sold at Sears among other places. Amplifon also owns Sonus. Altogether, according to a 2009 report in *Hearing Health*, the company owned 2800 retail outlets, and was affiliated with another 2000 shops and 3000 service centers.

Beltone, if not the largest, may be the most visible of the retail outlets, probably because the company's offices are usually freestanding and often in small towns. Beltone (again, in 2009) had 1400 affiliated outlets across the country. It's been in business for over sixty years.

Costco, despite having hearing aid centers in only 200 stores, is nevertheless the fourth-largest retailer in the country. Costco distributes Rexton hearing aids. Plans in 2009 to partner with AARP apparently fell through. That year AARP set up a partnership instead with HearUSA, another hearing care provider.

Sam's Club has also gotten into the hearing aid business, partnering with General Hearing Instruments, Inc.

The Veterans Administration has been a major distributor of hearing aids, propping up the whole hearing aid industry. In 2010,

VA purchases accounted for 24 percent of hearing aid sales for the year. This trend is slackening, however, in part because looser eligibility requirements allowed many veterans not previously entitled to hearing aids to get them, and the VA has now accommodated most of them. As previously noted, however, the wars in Iraq and Afghanistan have created a tremendous need for hearing aids among servicemen, despite the use of protective ear equipment.

Demographics alone suggest that the hearing aid business can only prosper. The number of people sixty-five and over is expected to nearly triple worldwide by 2050, according to a 2011 report from the Census Bureau. The worldwide sixty-five-plus population in 2011 was 545 million. Projections indicate that number will increase to 1.55 billion by 2050. Among these, the number of people with age-related hearing loss is expected to number 900 million.

VOICES: ROBERT ASTLE

Being a chef doesn't seem like a career that would be incompatible with hearing loss. But even without Led Zeppelin as background music, a restaurant kitchen is very noisy: bare surfaces, the clatter of dishes and the shouting of cooks and waiters, the equipment (exhaust hoods, washing machines), and colleagues with strong accents.

Toward the end of his cooking career, Robert Astle spent seven and a half years as a pastry chef in a Florida retirement facility. It was already difficult because of his hearing loss, but in 1998 he was diagnosed with type 2 diabetes as well. Now it was not only the noise but also the sugar and carbohydrates that threatened his health. In 2010, he broke a bone in his left foot, the result of poor blood sugar control, and was told not to expect to work in a standing position more than four hours a day. It was time for a new career, and, as he wrote to me, "a new chapter in my life."

Robert Astle (pronounced As-til), forty-six years old, was born with progressive hearing loss, probably caused by antibiotics his mother took during her pregnancy. Among the remedies his doctors tried were niacin pills, which caused him to flush, sweat a lot, and occasionally get hives. For a school-age child already having trouble fitting in because of hearing loss, these physical problems only added to his discomfort.

At thirteen, he got a hearing aid, which gave him "a big boost of confidence." Unlike many, he was "proud to show off" his hearing aid. "It gave me something to talk about," he said. "I don't remember that it gave me much of a boost in hearing, though."

Working in the kitchen, he had stopped wearing his hearing aids in 2006: "They only made sounds louder, not clearer," he said. "I heard a daily jumble of sounds. Struggling to lip-read, to watch body language and follow the context of conversations, I was exhausted at the end of the day." In 2008, he got a cochlear implant in his right ear.

His was not one of the "miracle" turn-on-day experiences. "My mother sat with me in the clinic room, and the CI was activated. Nothing happened." Nothing happened for three months, and even when it did, the implant was not much use to him. Three and a half years after implantation, his hearing with the implant tested at only 56 percent.

Nevertheless, in December of 2011 he got a second implant, like the first an Advanced Bionics model. He was one of the first recipients of Advanced Bionics' new Neptune implant, a waterproof device that can be clipped to a shirt collar, worn on a headband or armband—with a wire that connects to the magnet on the head, which contains the microphone. His experience with the second implant, he wrote, was "100,000 percent different. I could hear people in the room clearly. It was amazing." He speculates that since he is left-handed, perhaps implanting his dominant ear was a factor.

Astle has relied on many mentors over the years of his hearing issues. One who helped him find a new career after he left cooking is Dr. Vyasa Ramcharan, a fellow resident of the Orlando area, who helped him set up a medical records business. Medical charts are scanned into a digital format, saving space in cramped medical offices, saving trees by reducing the use of paper, and providing an easily accessible record for doctors and patients.

Astle is now in a position to give back, and he works as a mentor for others with hearing loss and for those considering getting a cochlear implant. "Sharing my experiences with others is very important for me, as others did for me when my time came." One lesson he shares: "I always find it easier to put yourself out there. The more you tell people about your situation, the better the communication."

EIGHT

Cyborg: Cochlear Implants

In late October of 2008, I finally went deaf. I was now profoundly deaf in my left ear, and able to hear in my right only with a new, stronger hearing aid, lipreading, and tremendous concentration.

That 2008 loss would prove to be fateful. Here's how it happened: I had a flu shot on a Monday, and Tuesday I felt dizzy and nauseated—the usual set of symptoms that signal a drop in my hearing. As always, I failed to recognize them, thinking (hoping? wishing?) it was a reaction to the shot. By Wednesday I was reeling. My hearing was supersensitive and the ground under my feet kept shifting. I was nauseated and from time to time retreated to the office restroom just to lean against the wall and breathe deeply until the nausea passed. I was able to hear almost nothing. I struggled through the week and on Friday went to see my otolaryngologist, Ronald Hoffman.

It was Halloween, and celebration had already begun by nine a.m., with kids and adults in costumes. The trip from my Upper West Side apartment (in rush hour) to the New York Eye and Ear Infirmary on Fourteenth Street and Second Avenue was surreal. The Ninety-sixth Street subway station was packed. It was hot. It was noisy beyond bearing. On the train, a panhandler in a wheelchair parked next to me to bellow his pitch, each word penetrating but incomprehensible. I shrank down in my seat, almost in a fetal position, to get away from the noise.

At New York Eye and Ear, in Dr. Hoffman's quiet office, he perched next to me on a rotating stool. I couldn't understand what he was saying. He reached for his laptop and typed his questions, turning the screen toward me. It was clear I had suffered a debilitating decline. He ordered some tests and wrote me a prescription for prednisone and a diuretic, part of the standard effort to reverse hearing loss. I'd taken them twice before, with little or no result. Neither of us expected it to work this time. It was a gesture. He'd see me again in two weeks.

The previous time I'd taken prednisone, a few years earlier after another drop in my hearing, I'd experienced a delirious high. I almost bought an apartment when I discovered that the penthouse in the building next door (which I can see from my windows) was on the market. My husband was doubtful, but I was unstoppable. Fortunately, at the last minute we were outbid. The apartment was way too small, but I still think of it longingly, and gaze out my own terrace-less windows at theirs.

This time the drug sent me reeling into depression. The psychiatrist I was already seeing (every person with hearing loss needs one) gave me a prescription for Klonopin, for anxiety, and her weekend telephone number. Three days of fear and anger, fighting with my husband, fighting with a store clerk, waking up at three in the morning and sitting on the bathroom floor in tears. On Sunday there was a minor work crisis that seemed major, especially because I had to deal with it on the phone, with several different people.

On Monday I went back to the office. I said I'd been out sick with the flu. Thus began the hardest year of my life, when I desperately pretended that I was a normal person, that I was a productive employee, that I could do it all.

Ten months later, I got a cochlear implant. It was only eight years after I had started with hearing aids. I resisted the idea of the implant, since I still had hearing in my right ear. But Dr. Hoffman pointed out that if the right ear went, I could be left with no hearing at all for months while I went through the implant process. Applying for insurance coverage for the procedure, going through the preliminaries (including a CT scan to rule out structural impediments to an implant), waiting for an opening in the surgeon's schedule—all these on their own could take many weeks. Once the surgery was completed, it would be another month before the implant could be activated, to allow the surgical wounds to heal. I reluctantly agreed, and began the screening procedure that spring. I had no choice about the date for the surgery, because of the doctor's schedule. The date was September 11. I was uneasy about being unconscious on the anniversary of 9/11, but the next available opening was months away.

One of the first steps in getting a cochlear implant is meeting with the audiologist at the implant center. Since Dr. Hoffman was at the cochlear implant center at New York Eye and Ear, I chose that hospital for the surgery. I was assigned to Megan Kuhlmey, tall and stolid, unflappable, a ready reassuring smile on her broad face. Megan would be my implant audiologist throughout all the preliminaries and afterward. She would continue to monitor my progress on a regular basis, reprogramming the implant as necessary. She would be my primary professional contact in the implant world, and she would prove to be a bulwark against flagging effort, discouragement, and impatience.

I now had two audiologists, one for each ear. Therese, slight, high-strung, frenetic, and Megan, tall, calm, and reassuring. Both acted as cheerleaders, confidantes, and colleagues in the effort to regain as much of my lost hearing as technology—and my own determination and hard work—would allow.

September 11, 2009, was horribly wet and rainy, nothing like that brilliant blue-sky day of September 11, 2001. Dan and I took the subway to New York Eye and Ear, at Fourteenth Street and Second Avenue, a familiar trip. But this time I went to Admitting, and soon was being asked dozens of questions, given a hospital gown and slippers, and shown to my room. It was only about nine a.m. and I knew the surgery wasn't scheduled till eleven, so I kept my street clothes on, reading and watching the deluge outside.

Finally a nurse told me I needed to put on the gown. Once I was dressed like a patient, I became a patient. I lay down on the bed. I got drowsy. The outside world, usually so insistent and demanding, seemed far away, not my concern.

Implant surgery is done on an outpatient basis, despite the room and bed and several hours under anesthesia. The surgery takes from one and a half to three hours and is getting shorter and more efficient all the time. But it's still a long day. I went in at eight in the morning and left the hospital at six, when I finally fully woke up from the anesthesia.

I wasn't able to watch the surgery, of course, but Michael Chorost describes the procedure in his book *Rebuilt: My Journey Back to the Hearing World.* His description is both technical and riveting. Although he is describing surgery on someone else, he writes as if it is being done on himself. Using a diamond-studded drill bit, he writes, the surgeon begins "excavating a tunnel in my mastoid bone toward my cochlea, which is buried an inch and a half deep inside my skull." The area where the drilling takes place, the skull base, is filled with dozens of blood vessels and nerves. Neurosurgeons often employ skull base surgeons to assist in getting through this area to the brain. In this case, however, the surgeon's drill would "travel within millimeters of my brain, but his target is my inner ear, not my cortex."

The cochlea is encased in a part of the temporal bone called the petrous bone. "You know the Greek root of 'petrous'?" Charles Liberman asked when I visited him at Harvard. "It's a stone. The petrous part of the temporal bone is the hardest bone in the body." The drill bit goes through this bone, exposing the cochlea. "So you've got this delicate little sensory structure with all these incredibly delicate hair cells encased in the hardest bone in the body, completely inaccessible," Liberman said. Completely inaccessible except with that drill bit. Very occasionally a surgeon will use the cochlea's natural opening, the round window, rather than drilling a hole in the bone of the cochlea.

It's a delicate operation with various opportunities for things to go wrong, but with an experienced surgeon they usually don't. Drilling the hole through the mastoid bone into the middle ear is routine for ear surgeons. The cochleostomy is a procedure only cochlear implant surgeons do. The facial nerve is a very close neighbor during this entire procedure—contact with it could cause partial paralysis of the muscles of the face. After the implant is inserted, the cochleostomy is sealed with body tissue, but cochlear fluid can leak out, causing balance problems.

Once the cochlea is exposed, Chorost writes, the surgeon blocks it with some gel foam as he moves to the area behind the ear where the body of the implant will go. "This part of the operation is pure carpentry: all he needs to do is create a well just deep enough so that the implant—about an inch square and the thickness of three quarters—will countersink neatly into my skull." After an examination of the implant itself under a microscope ("the electrode array leaps into sharp and enormously magnified focus"), the operation comes to its climax with the insertion of the electrode array into the cochlea.

How to insert the electrode array, less than an inch long, into the spiral of the cochlea was a problem that vexed researchers for more than forty years. It was Graeme Clark, a surgeon in Australia, who found the solution. "One day, when he was at the beach in Australia," Chorost writes of Clark, "he picked up a spiral-shaped shell and idly began poking grass stems into it, working the problem in his mind. After a while, he discovered that certain kinds of grass, which were stiff at the stem but flexible at the tip, slid smoothly into the shell without so much as cracking. That was it! *Differential stiffness!*"

The electrode array is inserted between twenty-five and thirty millimeters, approximately an inch and a half, into about one and a half rotations in the cochlea. The electrodes that go deepest into the cochlea serve the lower frequencies. Those in the shallowest part of the insertion (the end of the tail) serve the higher frequencies.

At Gallaudet University I saw a video of the insertion of the electrodes, one or two millimeters at a time, into the spiral cochlea. It was hard not to think of a very skilled Roto-Rooter operation.

My implant surgeon was Darius Kohan. Dr. Kohan is a colleague of Dr. Hoffman's and was in my health plan; by choosing him I thought the insurance plan might more quickly approve the surgery. Dr. Kohan had treated me earlier in the year in a last-ditch effort to restore my hearing with a procedure that involved injecting steroids directly into the ear, through the eardrum. It's just as unpleasant as it sounds. You lie on your side on an examining table, the ear to be treated facing up. My husband had come to the appointment with me, but he left the room once he saw the needle. After the injection you continue to lie on your side, the affected ear up so that nothing will spill out of it. You are told not to swallow for half an hour, to avoid egress by way of the eustachian tube, which connects to the throat. Try that sometime. The average person swallows about two thousand times a day. Try not swallowing for just a minute. One long drool. My husband was constantly handing me fresh paper towels.

The implant surgery, or at least my awareness of it, was tidy and painless by comparison. When I woke up, my head was swathed in a bandage that made me look like a refugee from *Swan Lake*. My ear and skull were bruised and tender, and I had a raw scar behind my ear that would take weeks to heal. The scar was small, two or three inches long, an improvement on early implant surgery, which left a big C-shaped scar across half the head. Dr. Hoffman, who assisted in the first multichannel implant on a child, in 1986, and began doing implant surgery on his own that year, described the old C incision as a huge flap that the surgeon would lift up to place the implant and electrode. Because the incision was so large, there was greater potential for infection or the edges of the scar corroding. The incisions have been getting smaller and smaller. If (when?) I get a second implant, the scar will be smaller than the first.

The implant itself, in my case a flat oval device the size of two quarters side by side, was placed under the skin about two inches northeast of my left ear. I can feel the outline of it under my hair. If I ever go bald, the implant will look like a flat plateau rising up from the landscape of my skull. After Dr. Kohan snaked the wire into my cochlea, connecting this minicomputer to my brain, he closed me up and sent me back to the room to sleep it off.

The hospital arranged for a car service to take us home. Shortly after I walked into the apartment, I was overcome by a wave of vertigo and nausea. That was not unexpected, and I'd been given meclizine (the antinausea drug sold commercially as Antivert) to help with the dizziness. I took one and slept for the next twelve hours. I continued to be dizzy for about three weeks, unsteady on uneven surfaces like the cobblestone walks along Central Park on upper Fifth Avenue.

Before the implant can be activated, the scars must have time to heal. This usually takes about a month. The wait for the implant to be "turned on" is an anxious time for many patients. Even though an audiologist has determined that the connection between the electrodes and the neurons has been made, there is no way to tell how well, or even if, the recipient will be able to hear. Will it work? What will I hear?

For those who have been deaf since birth, any sound at the point of activation can seem miraculous. For a formerly hearing person, the sound coming into the ear initially is just noise. No matter how modest your expectations, the moment can be deeply disappointing. The processor is now receiving sound digitally, turning it into a stream of bits (1s and 0s) and, via the electrodes connecting to the auditory nerves, transmitting them as radio waves to the brain. But within minutes, as the audiologist works with the preset programming, making adjustments on her computer, the noise begins to resolve into recognizable sound. With luck and practice, the brain will learn to hear the sounds as words, and the noise as the recognizable whoosh and clatter and rustle of everyday life.

On turn-on day and at regular visits afterward, Megan would

sit at her computer and reprogram my implant, guided by my answers to questions about how good the sound quality was. With preverbal children, this is not an option. Audiologists measure response based on the infant's facial movements and other physical signs. They're quite practiced at it, but it's not as accurate as an adult patient saying "That's too loud" or "I hear a hissing noise" or "I can hear you but I can't understand you."

. . .

John Oghalai at Stanford has been developing a technique that would allow audiologists to monitor the speech processes in a newly implanted deaf child, giving audiologists the same kind of information they receive aurally from adults. The most common imaging technique used to measure human brain function is the fMRI (functional Magnetic Resonance Imaging). Unfortunately, the magnetic components of the cochlear implant rule out MRI imaging unless the magnet is surgically removed.

Oghalai has been experimenting with a noninvasive neuroimaging technique called near-infrared spectroscopy (NIRS). The equipment is quiet and has no known risks, and is ideal for use in children with cochlear implants. In a 2010 study, he and his colleagues compared the results of speech-evoked brain activity in children with cochlear implants, by means of NIRS, with similar activity in hearing adults and hearing children by means of fMRIs.

Testing with unsedated small children has certain problems. The children, being children, can be squirmy or sleepy or cranky. "If a participant wished to take a break, cried, fell asleep for at least 30 seconds, or moved so much that the probes affected data collection, the session was terminated, and that participant's data were not included in the study. A typical NIRS testing session took ~20 minutes to complete." In all, 69 percent of the subjects completed the test.

NIRS, the authors of a study in *Hearing Research* concluded, could be useful in assessing the auditory function of deaf children using cochlear implants. The goal of this research is to make it possible to measure more accurately brain responses that would allow researchers and audiologists to improve speech and language skills in young implanted children. It is sometimes difficult to determine whether a preverbal child really is deaf before going ahead with a cochlear implant. The NIRS technology could be used in that situation as well.

An interesting unanticipated observation was that in deaf children with a new cochlear implant, brain responses appeared to be localized to the hemisphere of the brain closest to the implant. Most of the implants were in the right ear and the brain responses occurred in the right hemisphere. Noting that their study group was small, the researchers suggested further studies of this phenomenon, which is opposite to what is found in a normal hearing person. "This finding of right-sided activation is in contrast to the normal adult finding of left-hemisphere dominant language," they wrote, adding that the finding "suggests that auditory brain development in deaf children may be altered by the lack of normal sensory input."

Visiting Oghalai at Stanford, I asked if I could see the NIRS scanner, and he said I could try it out if I wanted. His lab is testing the technique on adults and they needed volunteers. With my cochlear implant and hearing aid, I made an ideal candidate. Oghalai introduced me to Homer Abaya, the research coordinator, who would perform the test. It would be repeated three times, once with the implant, once with the hearing aid, and once with neither. Fifteen minutes each.

Homer fitted a large headband around my head, which would transmit low-power near-infrared light beams through my scalp and skull and then measure the absorption of the light rays in the cerebral cortex. Over the headband he put a woolen cap, to help keep out ambient light. (I did wonder how many other heads had worn that hat.) Then, with me wearing the cochlear implant and the headband, he played a series of recorded sounds—voices reading, a cat meowing, hammering—for fifteen minutes. This was repeated with the hearing aid, and then with neither. The NIRS recorded the data, which would be analyzed to see how well I was hearing in all three situations.

. . .

Cochlear implants are indeed a miraculous device, restoring hearing to people who would otherwise live out their lives in silence. What the implant—and the brain—cannot do, however, is restore your hearing to the way it used to be. Cochlear implants are a tremendous advance for people with hearing loss. But as Stefan Heller and his colleagues, also at Stanford, wrote in a paper about patients' expectations and health care professionals' roles, "Cochlear implants and hearing aids are not perfect." Except for patients who are implanted in the first years of their life, "the efficacy of the devices vary substantially with regard to frequency discrimination, [and] performance in noisy environments, as well as simple day-by-day tasks such as speaking on the telephone."

Implants will improve: "Less invasive electrode placement and more highly selective spatial and temporal neural stimulation (whether electrical, optical, or chemical) offer considerable promise." But no matter how advanced these devices become, the paper went on, they are not likely to be a "cure" for hearing loss. "Problems inherent to all implantable devices will persist to some degree, including surgical risks, device failure, infection, and unfavorable tissue reactions . . . We will still not restore the entirely 'normal' perception that is so important to our patients with hearing loss."

But, as with hearing loss itself, I had no choice. Imperfect hearing or, possibly, no hearing at all. I was a cyborg, as Michael Chorost put it in *Rebuilt*. Not quite the Terminator, but nevertheless a being enhanced by artificial robotic parts. "An artificial sense organ makes your body literally someone else's," Chorost mused, "perceiving the world by a programmer's logic and rules instead of the ones biology and evolution gave you." Perhaps you need a programmer's mind to feel that way. For me, the implant is more like a prosthesis, something that allows me to function physically by artificial means.

The FDA first approved multichannel cochlear implants in 1984, initially on adults only. As of December 2010, about 71,000 Americans—42,600 adults and 28,400 children—now have at least one implant, according to the FDA. It is generally accepted that implants could benefit 250,000 Americans. Worldwide, the number of implants in 2010 was 219,000. Until recently, implants were approved only for those who were profoundly deaf, either from birth or as the result of accident or illness in midlife. Current FDA requirements are flexible, and implant centers can push a lot of envelopes. Medicare may balk at paying for implants that fall outside FDA guidelines, but private insurers rarely do. As implants get better and better, the FDA guidelines are continually expanded.

Three companies are licensed to sell implants in the United States: Cochlear, based in Australia; MED-EL, based in Austria; and Advanced Bionics, based in California. Cochlear was the first to be approved by the FDA. Within two years the lower age limit began to include younger and younger children. The three brands offer very similar features, and none is considered "better" than the others. The Cochlear Nucleus has twenty-two electrodes, which send the impulses to the auditory nerve system; MED-EL has twelve electrodes, and Advanced Bionics sixteen. The number is fairly irrelevant. "Users of all three systems are probably operating on four to eight electrodes," says Geoff Plant, who works with hearing-impaired people at the nonprofit Hearing Rehabilitation Foundation in Somerville, Massachusetts, two days a week, and for MED-EL another four.

Blake S. Wilson and Michael F. Dorman, writing in John Niparko's *Cochlear Implants: Principles and Practices*, concur. An important goal in implant design, they write, is to "maximize the number of largely non-overlapping populations of neurons that can be addressed by the electrode array. Present evidence suggests, however, that no more than four to eight independent sites are available using current speech processors and contemporary electrode designs, even for arrays with as many as twenty-two electrodes."

Every cochlear implant includes a microphone to pick up sound from the environment and a speech processor, which transforms the input from the analog world into a radiofrequency signal. The speech processor, which ordinarily sits behind the ear, contains the microphone, and is connected by a thin exterior cable to a disk about the size of a quarter that attaches magnetically to the implanted receiver. The receiver decodes the radiofrequency signal and sends the information down the implanted cable and into the cochlea, where the electrode array stimulates the neurons that send the signal to the auditory cortex. With luck, the cortex will hear it as identifiable sound.

Choosing between the three manufacturers is a little like throwing dice. Some hospitals or surgeons prefer one manufacturer or another, but I was given three large packets of information and told to take them home and decide what I liked best. I looked at the manufacturers' websites, read rapturous testimonials from users. But an implant is not something that you try one brand of and then switch to another. Each of these users had experience with only their own brand. Each brand claimed the best speech comprehension; the best musical fidelity, ease of use, etc.

Cochlear America is the largest seller in this country. I chose Advanced Bionics, for a frivolous reason: it had the sleekest external design. What I didn't know, but which turned out to be fortuitous, is that Advanced Bionics is the only manufacturer that offers a body-worn processor in addition to the much more common ear-level processor. This would turn out to be crucial to my use of the implant.

Unlike hearing aid manufacturers, cochlear implant companies flaunt their designs. Their brochures show their products on a model's head, fully visible. Taking the opposite tack from hearing aid manufacturers, implant manufacturers have started including multiple choices for the headpiece in all sorts of colors and psychedelic patterns. My current cover is blue, for no particular reason. I love seeing the kids with implants at the cochlear implant center, apparently completely oblivious of the earpiece and headpiece.

Cochlear implants can be more or less successful, depending on the user. But two factors are clear predictors of success. The first, for a child, is age. Implant surgery is far more successful if it's done when the child is still prelingual. These days children are implanted as young as six months, though different implant centers differ in the youngest ages. As Dr. Hoffman said, "The earlier the better," though one problem with very early implanting is ascertaining that the infant is in fact deaf. At Hopkins, Niparko said, they implant children beginning at eight months. They feel the extra two months helps reduce the danger of infection.

In adults, the most important factor is the length of time between losing the hearing and getting the implant. The more recently the hearing has been lost, the more likely it is that the implant will work well. In adults, age seems to be irrelevant. The oldest patient Dr. Hoffman has implanted, he told me, was ninety. Because implant surgery is so noninvasive, it's much less difficult for an older person than surgery on the chest, the bowel, even the elbow. With elbow surgery an older person may end up with phlebitis from no movement. Chest surgery can lead to pneumonia. For implant surgery, he said, "If the person is in any kind of decent physical shape, it's just not that invasive." Of course, he added, most people's definition of a big operation is any operation done on them. Implant surgery felt like a big operation to me.

Hopkins, with a full-time implant team of five implant surgeons, does about 260 surgeries a year, half on children, half on adults. New York Eye and Ear, with four full-time implant surgeons (and several others, like Dr. Kohan, who are affiliated with the hospital), does about 130 surgeries a year, also with half of them on children. About 40 percent are Medicaid patients. New York State has a relatively good Medicaid program. Other states have much greater restrictions on implant surgery. Arizona, Dr. Hoffman said, won't even pay for a liver transplant.

Programs like Arizona's are a false economy, Dr. Hoffman went on. We were talking in his office at the implant center, on Twenty-second street and Second Avenue, which he had helped establish and which is still affiliated with New York Eye and Ear but in a different building. He jumped up from his chair and took me down the hall to meet Brendan Vasanth, an adorable, scruffy-haired four-year-old who had gotten his first implant at eight months and his second at eleven months. His younger sister, Kate, was implanted at six months and nine months.

Brendan and Kate's mother, Lisa, is a doctor herself (a rheumatologist), and hearing. Brendan was working with a speech pathologist and his eyes lit up as we came into the room. Dr. Hoffman introduced me to Brendan and his mother and then chatted with Brendan, asking what he most likes about school (playground). As we left, Brendan gave Dr. Hoffman a high five. He gave me one too. It was difficult with my own hearing loss to hear how well he spoke, but Dr. Hoffman said that Brendan speaks perfectly. Lisa Vasanth said that other parents and kids at his school often don't even realize he has hearing loss.

Implants for children like Brendan save the state far more than the cost of the implant itself. "The sad thing is, it's stupid," Dr. Hoffman said. "There are lots of studies that show if you take a child like Brendan and implant him early, you save 400,000 dollars in education costs, through grade twelve. Yet the savings to the state for education goes into a silo that is totally separate from the medical costs. We need better reimbursement for the services provided to children, but we can't get beyond the separate 'silo' problem."

And you give the child a life as well. With hearing parents (90 percent of deaf children have hearing parents), Brendan and Kate would have a hard time being part of the Deaf community even if they and their parents became fluent in sign language. Without implants, a child like Brendan would be encased in silence, dependent on others as links to the hearing world. In school he would need an interpreter, unless he went to a school for the deaf. In that case he would need an interpreter to manage in the outside hearing world.

• • •

The adult brain has approximately 100 billion nerve cells, each with specific identities and patterns of neural connections. Some of these nerve cells and neuronal connections are genetically specified, but since mammals have 100,000 genes and the brain has 10^{15} neural connections, obviously the genes are outnumbered. The brain relies on environmental triggers to activate different subsets of genes at different periods of development. These triggers include nutrition, sensory and social experiences, and learning.

Brain cells continue to be produced until shortly after birth. In humans, no new neurons are thought to be created after the age of two or three, according to Charles J. Limb of Johns Hopkins, though basic neural connections continue to be made until the late teenage years. But it is during early development that the plasticity of the brain is at its maximum, and the most important factor for proper development of the brain—and of the auditory system—is stimulation. In a hearing child, that stimulation comes through sound. But in deaf children, the brain is able to utilize these same areas of the cortex (deprived of input in the form of sound) for other purposes.

"The brain is remarkably capable of extracting useful information from seemingly sparse input," write Dr. Limb and his Johns Hopkins colleague David K. Ryugo. "It follows, then, that the stimulation received by the auditory system need not be acoustic in nature." Electrical stimulation, provided by cochlear implants, allows the developing child to learn to associate visual, somatosensory, and other environmental clues with the electrical signal coming from the implant. This works best when the brain is still devoid of information that may already have begun to form neural pathways. A child who has learned sign language or a severely hearing-impaired child who has learned some minimal speech will have to retrain the brain to recognize those electrical signals as representing sound, to reprocess their auditory pathways. Up till age three or four the brain remains relatively plastic, and most implant surgeons prefer to implant before this age.

Early studies indicated that children with cochlear implants did markedly better than their signing peers in standardized academic tests. The children tested had mostly been implanted no earlier than the age of three, and many up till the age of seven. Early testing found improvement in reading scores for the implanted group, but in later testing (as the children with implants began to reach middle and high school) the results dropped off.

A comprehensive 2007 review article published in the *Journal of Deaf Studies and Deaf Education* attempted to sort out the seemingly conflicting results from a number of studies. The article noted that a variety of recent studies had demonstrated benefits to hearing, language, and speech from implants, "leading to assumptions that early implantation and longer periods of implant should be associated with higher reading and academic achievement." Their review, however, found more nuanced results: "Although there are clear benefits of cochlear implantation to achievement in young deaf children, empirical results have been somewhat variable."

After discussing each of the studies, the authors addressed the implications of the findings. First, though, they noted the importance of looking at academic achievement more broadly than simply by comparing standardized test scores. Cochlear implants fall short of providing deaf children with classroom information that is available to their hearing peers. The seeming "obsession" of educators and investigators with deaf children's literacy skills ignores other challenges across the curriculum.

One of the authors they cite suggested that "cochlear implants may work too well." Teachers think children with implants are hearing normally and don't need extra support services in the classroom. But a classroom is typically a noisy place, and while children with implants may hear what is said to them directly, they miss much else that contributes to a broad academic and social knowledge. By the time they reach high school, deaf children may have excellent intelligibility of speech but lack "the sophisticated language to deal with complex curricula, particularly in noise and with changing teachers."

These findings may change as the database for children implanted early begins to grow. So far, no studies have looked at children implanted before one year, which implant surgeons agree is optimal. That group of children is just beginning to reach middle and high school age. The studies that do exist compare children implanted at age three or later, but even these studies find that the younger the age of implantation, the better on average the academic performance.

Finally, the review authors note that in all the studies, children were implanted at a later period than they are now. "It remains to be seen whether similar findings are obtained with children who are implanted within the first year." They clearly have their doubts: "Given the findings thus far, however, one should not assume that academic differences between deaf children and their hearing peers will disappear."

Cochlear implants remain controversial in the proud and tightly knit Deaf community. A wrenching documentary, *Sound and Fury*, directed by Josh Aronson, follows two families with both Deaf and hearing members as two adult brothers and their wives and their extended family debate whether to get their deaf children implanted. The movie was released in 2000, but the issues remain contemporary. Passions run high, especially among the Deaf, who see their culture threatened.

Hurtful things are said: "Look, if she doesn't want the baby because he's deaf, I'll take him," says the Deaf grandmother. "My friends wonder why she won't love her own child, even if he's born deaf," another Deaf relative says. "A mother should love her child the way he is."

Leah Hager Cohen grew up as a hearing child in the Lexington School for the Deaf (her parents both worked there), understanding both sign and spoken language. Her beautifully written book *Train Go Sorry*, now a classic of Deaf literature, is an intimate look at the lives of students with hearing loss. The Lexington School had been founded in the oralist tradition—deaf children were to wear hearing aids and speak, using lipreading and other aids, including early FM devices. As noted elsewhere, the majority of "deaf" people have some degree of hearing, and the children at the Lexington School mostly benefited from their hearing aids. Learning to speak would better prepare them for the outside world, the oralists maintained, and sign language was not allowed in the classroom.

The students did sign in private, so Cohen grew up with both spoken language and sign. As she explains, echoing the observations in the review paper, the deaf child hears the essentials but does not pick up the asides, the nuances that create a more comprehensive embrace of the culture and that contribute to a more expanded vocabulary. "I was constantly absorbing the banter between teacher and assistant, picking up new vocabulary, cadences and constructions," she writes. "The others were not."

Even with all the technology available to the deaf today, Cohen writes, socially, there is still the need for a place for the deaf to be together. "All these modern developments have done little to quench deaf people's thirst for time spent physically together. When so much of the world is indecipherable, so much information inaccessible, the act of congregating with other deaf people and exchanging information in a shared language takes on a kind of vital warmth." There are very few schools for the deaf remaining. Most deaf children are mainstreamed in public schools. I wonder if they feel that thirst for time spent physically together with others like them.

One place where that physical togetherness still exists is at Gallaudet University, which maintains an ASL-only tradition among faculty, students, and staff. Visiting Gallaudet as a hearing person without knowledge of sign language, as I did in 2011 for a conference, was like stepping into a country where I not only didn't understand the language but couldn't even read the alphabet. All around me, students were in animated conversation; I saw a group practicing for a performance, laughing and shouting and creating a terrible din but never uttering a word. I expected a hushed campus and instead found one alive with sound. But no spoken language. And interestingly, since I was staying in a conference center hotel open to the public, no written signs to help the hearing navigate.

The morning I arrived, I went to meet my group in the designated room off the café, where we had been told lunch would be provided for free. While waiting, I went to the coffee machine, and since I planned to drink the coffee while I looked around, I took a paper cup. Suddenly the cashier was at my side, gesticulating, at first impatiently and then angrily, about my choice of coffee cups. I had no idea what the issue was until someone later told me that the coffee was free only if you used a ceramic cup. For paper you had to pay. A simple sign would have saved a lot of wasted energy on the cashier's part, and confused humiliation on mine.

This is how the hard of hearing often feel in the hearing world, although public facilities increasingly are installing visual devices to aid people with hearing loss. Until very recently, announcements on the New York subway system were made through an unintelligible (even to the fully hearing) public address system. In the past few years, LED displays have been set up everywhere, informing riders about delays, route changes, and even when the next train is arriving. New York has finally caught up with all the other cities around the world that have been using LED displays for years.

• • •

There is one group for whom cochlear implants are not advised (though they are not prohibited from getting them). Implanting a prelingually deaf adult, experts agree, "does not have satisfactory results," as Ryugo and Limb bluntly put it. The family of a deaf child may decide when the child is a teenager that some hearing would be useful, Elizabeth Ying, the director of Hearing

Habilitation at my implant center, told me. Requesting an implant, they say that they want to give their teenage child a sense of place. "We really only want him to be able to hear when he's riding his bike down the street." She said, "On the hookup day, they expect him to be able to talk on the phone."

The difficulty of adjusting to an implant as an adult who has never heard spoken language was poignantly demonstrated in the 2007 HBO documentary *Hear and Now*. The filmmaker, Irene Taylor Brodsky, follows her parents, both sixty-five and deaf for their entire lives, as they decide upon retirement to get cochlear implants. They go through a minimal screening process and are approved for the procedure.

Happily active in the Deaf community, the parents of four loving children, Brodsky's parents are devastated by the implant experience. The bewildered parents, especially the mother, can't comprehend what they're hearing. Eventually the mother gives up using the implant. Her husband continues with it, but essentially both go back to the silent life they know. It's a sweet, touching film, a bold, difficult experiment seen through a loving daughter's eyes.

Ryugo and Limb hold out the possibility that implants in people like the Taylors may be successful in the future: "With further research," they write, "the mature brain may some day be sufficiently understood such that language skills can be acquired by prelingually deafened adults as easily as they are by normal children."

Although I am in the second most promising category for implantees (adults who have only recently lost their hearing), my mature brain has had a difficult time reacquiring language skills. My left ear, the implant ear, had been relatively nonfunctional for thirty years when I got the implant, though I had lost all hearing only the year before. Thus the neural pathways for language had received little stimulation and were atrophying. The longer the period between the onset of deafness and the implant, the less plasticity the auditory neural pathways have retained. In addition, my neural pathways were trained to hear acoustically. Now they were not only being asked to function again, but to function in a different way than they once did.

Probably the greatest detriment to my success with the implant was the timing. My implant was turned on in October of 2009. The months of October, November, and December, when I left the *Times*, were a period of intense personal and professional turmoil. I wore the implant, but I made little effort to train myself to hear with it. Those first three months are crucial and should be filled with rehabilitative work, either with a speech language pathologist (which is routine for children but not adults) or through the many interactive programs offered online. I signed on to the Advanced Bionics "Listening Room" but was quickly deterred when I discovered that the CLIX program (a central piece of their rehab software) was not available on Apple computers. I didn't seriously start rehab until almost six months after implantation. And that was too late.

• • •

An earlier start would not have helped with the enjoyment of music. Cochlear implants are designed to maximize comprehension of speech. So far, comprehension—and enjoyment—of music lies far behind.

Charles Limb is an associate professor in the department of Otolaryngology–Head and Neck Surgery at Johns Hopkins, a musician, and a member of the faculty at the Peabody Conservatory of Music. His interest in music and the brain is wide-ranging: in a recent TED talk (available online) he spoke about preliminary studies of the brain on music. Limb monitored the jazz pianist Mike Pope as he underwent a functional MRI, flat on his back with a miniature computerized piano in his lap, allowed to move only his hands. Limb in the control room with a keyboard and Pope in the MRI machine improvised. Describing the experience, Pope said, "There were moments, for sure, of honest-to-God musical interplay." What the fMRI showed was that the *language* areas of Pope's brain, the Broca's area—"the areas of expressive communication"—as Limb put it, lit up. "This whole idea that music is a language, well maybe there's a neurological basis to it after all."

I met with Limb at Hopkins in the spring of 2011, to talk about music and cochlear implants, two subjects that don't usually belong in the same sentence—as implant users know. There is no such thing as "music" for someone with a cochlear implant. Limb commented that what the cochlear implant companies do now, in terms of music, is try to adapt technology designed for speech. People with implants can generally hear rhythm, but very few can hear pitch. "Once pitch is distorted it is very hard to understand melody, because melody is based on pitch intervals.

"There is nothing harder to hear than music," he went on. "Music is the most complex auditory stimulus there is. Because it's so difficult acoustically, it's going to be really hard for an implant." Another researcher had said that perfecting the ability to hear music was the holy grail of implant research.

Limb pointed out that a second factor affecting the ability to hear music is lack of context: "Language has semantics, okay, so even if the sound quality of my voice to you is poor, if you can understand what I'm saying you kind of get it. In music there is no 'What was he saying?'" to provide context. "Musically, there's no clear meaning. So the impact of that music on you, which is subjective, can't be measured." There is no objective test, as there is in measuring speech perception with an implant. All we can ask is "How did it affect you?

"It's devastating to many musicians," Limb continued. I had heard this directly from the musicians I interviewed, over and over again. Not only could they not perform but they could not enjoy music. "There are very few people with implants that were really, really high-level musicians, and very few of those that can still hear music well, very few." Interesting preliminary studies have shown that children implanted early tested almost as well as hearing children on the ability to hear pitch intervals, rhythm, timbre, melo-dies, and harmony, but there have not been follow-up tests as they aged.

• • •

Almost three years after my implant, I was still relying heavily on my hearing-aided ear, and I continued to have a great deal of diffi-culty with the vowel sounds. Bit or bet; prim or prom; lift, left, loft, laughed. They're all one to me.

Relearning to hear is in many ways similar to long-term psycho-therapy, especially psychoanalytically based therapy. Studies have shown that talk therapy, as well as antidepressants and other medica-tions, actually changes the neural pathways over time. The time I have spent trying to change the neural pathways in my auditory sys-tem has overlapped with the time I have spent trying to change the neural pathways that regulate emotional behavior. Those pathways—which resulted in depression, anger, anxiety—were as deeply en-trenched as the auditory neural pathways that had come to recognize language only in the form of sound. I imagine my brain sometimes, when I let my vigilance down, shooting off electrical connections down the old pathways, breaking through the fragile barriers like a car crashing through a sawhorse barricade onto an old road. I have to back up, set the barricade up again, and consciously turn down the new route, whether it is the newly formulated auditory pathway or the new emotional pathway. Both are still freshly paved, sticky, throwing up bits of gravel. But eventually, I hope, they'll smooth out, solidify, become the easier way to go.

For me, a cochlear implant was a last resort. But as standards for implantation relax, and as the surgery becomes increasingly safe and minimal, implants have become the treatment of choice for many. Ryan M. Carpenter writes that although neither hearing aids nor cochlear implants mimic acoustic hearing, implants can be a more successful alternative for those with sensorineural hearing loss. "With training and practice, most recipients describe the sound quality of their cochlear implant(s) as clearer, sharper, and more comfortable than that of hearing aids."

VOICES: LORIE SINGER

Lorie Singer works at the Cochlear Implant Center at New York Eye and Ear and seems to be the go-to person for everything, though officially she is Technical Services Coordinator. She has one cochlear implant and is considering getting another, but I wouldn't have known she had any hearing difficulty if she hadn't told me.

I see Lorie almost every time I go to the implant center, but one day we sat down in her office for an interview. She has an M.B.A. in business management and an undergraduate degree in biology. Her background led her naturally to medical publishing, where she was working when her hearing went. She couldn't hear the phone ring, she said, and finally made an appointment with an audiologist. "How do you get through the day?" the audiologist asked sympathetically. "I burst into tears," Lorie said. Someone finally recognized what she was going through. A hearing aid in her left ear enabled her to keep working until she was thirty-nine. At that point, once again unable to use the telephone, she felt she had to leave the job.

"I was really frustrated," she said. "I was ready to kill someone." As with many New Yorkers, her first stop was the League for the Hard of Hearing. Dorene Watkins, an audiologist, told her she needed a cochlear implant. "But I'm not deaf," Lorie responded. Classic denial. Her hearing loss is genetic. Her grandmother was deaf by the time she was forty. Both her mother and her sister have hearing loss.

Dr. Hoffman, then at NYU, did Lorie's surgery in 1996. The procedure was more major than it is now, involving a larger incision, called a Lazy J. (That incision replaced the *C* incision, which basically opened up a flap of skin the size of your palm.) She had the surgery on a Wednesday, spent the night in the hospital, and went back to work the following Monday. NYU suggested she wait six months for auditory rehab, but she started after three months. "I pursued it on my own, at the League for the Hard of Hearing." Her initial experience with the implant was difficult, but, she said, "I had no choice but to learn to use it. It was totally horrible at first. But now Paul McCartney sounds like Paul McCartney."

She also worked with Books on Tape, reading along with them. "A lot of hard-of-hearing people develop a life where they don't talk to people, even after they get the implant. Even though it wasn't my job, I'd make all kinds of suggestions. Go to a lecture, go to Barnes and Noble to a reading, listen to Books on Tape.

"My expectation was that the cochlear implant would give me a little better sound," she said. "But it's better than that." Still, she cautions people not to expect too much. "People who have more hearing loss do better, are more appreciative. People with less, people who come in and say they want one because they want to be able to use the phone a little better, they're more likely to be disappointed."

For someone as no-nonsense as Lorie is, she is surprisingly hesitant about getting a second implant despite the benefits she would get from binaural hearing. "The reason I haven't gotten it?" she said. "It's going to take a lot of work to get used to it. I'm not sure I want to do that again. I'm very focused. I would want to get everything I could out of it. And I can hear fine with one ear."

In the end, we talked as much about me as about her. She was full of practical advice. Was I using the phone device? She gave me one. She's right. It's amazing. I bought two new phones the very first day (the dial has to be on the body of the phone, not the handset, for the cochlear implant connection). I hear on my hearing aid side through the handset and on the implant side through the attached device. Binaural hearing on the phone!

NINE

Wig Tape, and That Pig Outdoors

Some people manage to look dignified wearing an implant. Not me.

For the first several months after my surgery and turn-on day in October 2011, I was prone to pratfalls, the earpiece constantly slipping off, dragging the silvery magnet with it, or the magnet itself becoming attracted to something besides the implant (an umbrella spoke, say), detaching itself and dragging the earpiece with it. If I brushed back my hair, or turned my head, or flipped up the collar of my jacket, or wrapped a scarf around my neck, or put on a hat, off went the earpiece, sometimes flying across the room. The magnet attracted anything in its vicinity. When I stepped into my closet, it pulled in the chain from the overhead light. If I was reading in bed and leaned back too close to the metal bed frame, the magnet popped off my head and stuck to the bed frame. If I put it down near a hearing aid battery, the battery leaped to connect itself to the implant magnet.

I started out with the standard adult implant apparatus. The processor in the brand I had, Advanced Bionics, is a handsome titanium curve the size of a large hearing aid—a mammoth hearing aid, if you're trying to keep it invisible—powered by a rechargeable battery that snaps onto it. It's designed to fit behind the ear. Mine perched rather than nestled. Michael Chorost described his behind-the-ear hearing aid as looking like a cat draped over a La-Z-Boy. My processor looked more like a cat precariously balanced on a window ledge. The battery, the size of one joint of a thumb, was supposed to hug the back of the ear, behind the earlobe. But my ears weren't made for nestling or hugging. They're small. And, as my audiologist put it, "floppy."

I do have floppy ears. But the real problem was that I didn't want to acknowledge the device—to myself, and especially not to anyone else. I did everything I could to hide it, and when it refused to stay hidden I scrambled furtively to cover up the evidence. If the earpiece fell off, I'd shove it in my pocket instead of putting it back behind my ear. I tugged and pulled at my hair in a futile attempt to keep the earpiece covered, which of course only made it or the magnet fall off. I tucked a small mirror into my pocket, and stepped into the ladies' room at every opportunity to check if the magnet was still screened by my hair, that the cable was lying flat instead of curling up as if I were being electrocuted, that the earpiece was hidden behind my ear. It rarely was. My ears were not big enough and my hair was not long enough. The squared-off end of the magnet could always be seen. I was all too eager to keep up the subterfuge and denial that I had hearing loss, but it was harder with a large piece of hardware behind my ear.

The wobbly earpiece wasn't the only problem. The magnet itself has to be strong enough to hold the implant in place but not so strong that the pull of it would damage the skin underneath. Megan Kuhlmey, my audiologist at the implant center, started me out with a fairly weak magnet. It fell off a lot, usually taking the earpiece with it. On one occasion, while I was cleaning the oven, magnet and earpiece fell way too close to a foamy puddle of Easy-Off. I was fearful it would fall into the toilet or onto the subway tracks.

The problems started on turn-on day—the moment when you hear again after years of deafness, or perhaps for the first time ever. I'd been invited to the opera that evening with a friend from the Culture department. The performance was *Der Rosenkavalier* with Renée Fleming, and I had been looking forward to it for weeks. Orchestra seats. Sold out. Tickets like this were the best perk of the

Culture department. In her office that afternoon, Megan urged me to wear the implant all the time, even to the opera that night. She preferred that I not wear the hearing aid as well as I got used to the implant, but I implored her. I needed to be able to hear. So I wore both, and still do.

That evening, I washed, fluffed, and sprayed my hair to make sure it stayed in place over the implant. My posture was perfect to the point of rigidity, so as not to tip it off. I locked my hands in my lap to ensure I didn't brush against my hair. Even so, midway through Act III, the implant got dislodged and dropped into my lap. Thank goodness it was *my* lap. Implants are designed to maximize voice sounds, and music is one of the areas where they are least helpful, as I would learn. I heard well enough with my hearing aid to make the evening enjoyable, though primarily on a visual level.

Over the next few weeks, I saw Megan regularly for reprogramming. On one visit she gave me a little plastic ear harness, something like a dog muzzle, that fit over my ear and the implant, holding it in place. Some days I wore a scarf to anchor the earpiece to my head, or a headband. I wrapped Band-Aids around the battery to make it less slippery and less visible. I went on the Advanced Bionics website and scrolled through comments to see if anyone else had this problem. One writer suggested moleskin. It didn't help. Then, at one of my regular appointments with Megan, she mentioned wig tape.

Wig tape is double-sided tape. Its primary purpose is just what it says—to hold a wig steady on your head. It's deviously tricky to expose both sides without getting your fingers stuck, or accidentally folding it onto itself. That night, after work, I went to Ricky's, the costume shop, running through drenching rain, determined not to wait another day to try it. It was almost Halloween and the store and its patrons were garishly surreal.

The next morning, I managed to expose both sides of the tape and glue it to the earpiece and its battery and then fit it behind my ear. Not only did it not fall off, it wasn't even visible. I was ecstatic. I also thought I was hearing better. But that night, when it came time to take it off, the tape ripped out the skin and hair that had gotten stuck to it. Painful. I never wore wig tape again, but it turned out to be great for installing shelf paper, getting cupboard doors to shut firmly, and holding a photo in place under a mat.

I was beginning to think I might just stop wearing the implant. Megan dug around in her drawer full of implant cable wires and new batteries and plastic harnesses, pulling out a clunky gray metal device about the size of a cell phone—or a pack of unfiltered Camel cigarettes—but heavier and less sleek. It was a body-worn processor. I could put it in my pocket and run the long cable under my shirt and up to the magnetized disk under my scalp.

The cable on the processor Megan lent me was intended for a child, someone four feet tall, and was too short to reach to my pocket or a belt. While I waited for the longer cable, I mostly wore the processor tucked in my bra, giving my left breast a squarish shape. But I could move my head without dislodging the whole apparatus and I felt liberated. The headpiece still tended to fly off, but it just dangled by the cable rather than dropping to the floor. The controls were on the box.

Fishing around inside my bra to change the volume and noise programs (one for quiet places, one for noisy ones) was problematic, but once I got a longer cable I could discreetly change the settings just by reaching into my pocket. By contrast, the ear-level processor, that devilish device, has its controls on the processor itself. To turn it up or down, you rotate a tiny dial with a thumbnail. Very hard to do without taking it off and looking at the dial. So mine was improperly set much of the time.

About three months after I got the implant, I was invited to lunch by Sue Grossman, a handsome woman some years older than me who had allowed *The New York Times* to write about her implant experience. We'd gotten in touch after the article appeared and met in a noisy restaurant where neither of us could hear a thing—she with her implants (one in each ear), me then with just a hearing aid. But we continued to correspond by e-mail. On this January day I headed over to York Avenue, about as far east as you can get in Manhattan, to her apartment. She and her husband, a real estate developer, had recently moved from Queens into Manhattan to be closer to New York culture. Shortly after the move, Sue's hearing had deteriorated so much that they gave up their Carnegie Hall subscription. But she still gamely got on the bus and went to museums and restaurants, with the enthusiasm of a new arrival.

Also at lunch was a woman named Judy, who was eighty-eight, fine-boned and elegant, and who had gotten an implant about three months before Sue did. They had met at NYU, where they both had their surgery. Despite her age and deafness, Judy still worked as a volunteer at the UN. She couldn't hear any better than I could but, like Sue, seemed delighted to be hearing at all. Sue had implants in both ears, Judy in just one, and neither had any trouble keeping them on their heads. They wore them with gratitude and flair. I felt like a curmudgeon.

Both Sue's and Judy's implants were made by the Cochlear Company. The Cochlear Nucleus seemed, in retrospect, as if it might be a little easier to wear. MED-EL's earpiece seemed a little bulkier. AB is sleek and silvery. The AB magnet comes with interchangeable metallic caps—iridescent colors or splashy patterns. Caucasian flesh color, in retrospect, would have been more discreet. Maybe that's why Sue and Judy seemed so much more comfortable with theirs. Or maybe the Cochlear is just a more flexible fit. It may also be slightly smaller. The magnet I have now is blue and always will be, since my dog got hold of it and mashed it permanently in position.

I had just gotten my new body-worn processor the day I went to Sue's for lunch. I wore jeans, with the processor in my pocket, the cable running up my back under my shirt. I was pleased with it, but Sue and Judy were appalled, mostly by the cable. "What if you want to wear a bathing suit?" Sue asked, as if that were a daily problem.

There *are* lots of things I can't wear, including slinky dresses and pants without pockets, but I was willing to sacrifice part of my wardrobe in order not to have to admit I was wearing an implant.

Eventually, in a runners' store, I found a belt for holding a cell phone while running. The processor fit perfectly. So now I wear the belt under a loose shirt or sweater if I don't have pockets. I also now wear the behind-the-ear processor more often, if I'm not doing anything too vigorous—like sports or housecleaning. It still falls off, but until the day it falls off into the toilet or onto the subway tracks, I can live with it.

In the winter of 2012, Advanced Bionics came out with a new processor, which could be used with my existing implant. Called a Neptune, it's also a body-worn processor, but it's a small device worn with a clip attached to a headband or a shirt collar, with a short wire connecting the magnet to the implant. It's also waterproof (hence the name). I would love to have one, but at a cost of $9000 to trade in my Platinum body-worn, I probably won't be getting one soon.

Two and a half years after my implant, I'm discovering that although the implanted receiver is meant to last for life, other components aren't. I'll need new batteries for both processors: $165 apiece for the Harmony behind-the-ear model and $99 apiece for the body-worn Platinum. You need at least two working batteries, since one charges while you use the other.

I have also snapped the cable of the body-worn several times. It's too long (42 inches—the next longest is too short, at 32 inches), and because it's too long it tends to snag on door handles and snap off—$43. Recently I impatiently threw the whole cable away after I snapped it on a door handle once again, and only later realized that I had also thrown away the headpiece that magnetically attaches to the implanted receiver—$350.

. . .

My vanity exasperated everyone. This all would have been easier if I'd been willing to acknowledge how hard it was for me to hear. And to wear my implant with pride. But I wasn't yet ready to acknowledge disability. I was far from alone in this attitude, as I was to discover.

I was still not doing well five or six months after the implant, and Megan suggested auditory therapy. She referred me to a program at the Center for Hearing and Communication (the old League for the Hard of Hearing). I went in for an evaluation. The center is at 50 Broadway, just around the corner from the Stock Exchange. Cars are banned from many streets, and Wall Street itself looks heavily fortified: barricades, police officers in full riot gear, dogs. Wandering around and through them are hordes of tourists, cameras at the ready.

The Shelley and Steven Einhorn Communication Center at the Center for Hearing and Communication serves a wide clientele, providing not just speech therapy and auditory training and speech-reading (what we used to call lipreading), but fitting and selling hearing aids as well. The waiting room was usually crowded with very old people, and younger people with severe disabilities in addition to their hearing loss. It was depressing. The implant center at NYEE, like the Communication Center, served a number of families on Medicaid, but the building was new and the afflicted in general were young children, whose natural buoyancy and curiosity gave that waiting room an energetic and often entertaining atmosphere. (I later learned that the Center for Hearing and Communication has a separate waiting room for children.)

The speech pathologist assigned to evaluate me for audiotherapy led me back to her office. Short, dumpy, wearing baggy pants with an elasticized waist and a fanny pack over her stomach, she had made the worst of her looks. She was disorganized, shuffled papers around, pushing aside a half-empty carton of apple juice and an open package of crackers; she didn't seem sure where anything was. The evaluation questions were ones I've been asked zillions of times—word recognition, sentence recognition. I told her the better hearing in my right ear made it difficult to judge how clearly I heard with the implant. She vaguely suggested white noise in the right ear and then seemed to forget about it. I held my hand over my ear, with the hearing aid muted, to try to keep the right ear from hearing. She was glacially slow; perhaps she was used to talking to the very old, or the feebleminded. I sank deeper and deeper into despair. I literally felt myself sinking in the chair. I went home feeling that I'd gone from being a competent professional to a hearing-impaired retiree.

When I was leaving, the therapist said she was sure I would qualify for their hearing rehabilitation program and that she would be happy to work with me. I groaned to myself. Later, I got up my nerve and asked the center if I could be assigned to a different therapist. I was given an appointment with Linda Kessler, the assistant director at the Einhorn Center. I liked her immediately. She was smart and businesslike, and we covered a lot of territory in my weekly hour-long sessions. That is not to say that I mastered the territory, just that we covered it.

• • •

A few weeks after I started, Linda Kessler and I stood looking at our faces in a mirror, studying the shape of our mouths as we pushed out a *p*.

"No," she said. "You're puckering your lips. Watch me. My lips are relaxed and just meeting. Let the air get out but don't use your voice." I watched. "P!"

Then it was my turn. "P!" Wrong. "Let's do it together," she said. We seemed to be doing exactly the same thing, except that her lipsticked lips, carefully made-up face, and tinted shiny auburn hair looked a lot better than my long, too thin, too pale, too depressed visage.

"Breath or voice?" she asked. I desperately tried to remember the practice sheet of letters divided into breath and voice, since I had no idea just by hearing it. I tried "breath." Yes!

Linda had been trying to teach me how to say the sound "p"—versus the name of the letter—for weeks. I kept saying "pea" and she wanted me to say just the "p" without a long *e* after it. Kind of like spitting.

In order to say it properly, I needed to know how the sound is made. Each consonant has three aspects. Is it made with breath or voice? What is the method of production (the only one of those I ever got was "plosive")? Where in the mouth is the sound made? I simply could not wrap my mind around this. Week after week she asked me the same questions, and week after week I got the answers wrong. After she'd told me three or four times over the weeks that most people get this concept easily, I quit. I couldn't afford the $125 a week anyway.

A year or so later, I went back to talk with her. I was interested in her approach. Why did she put so much emphasis on the physiological formation of sounds? Linda looked as well coifed and carefully made up as ever, but there was a sense of anxiety, of distraction, that I hadn't seen before. She had a project to report, she said, and had more work to do on it, so we'd have to talk quickly. Later she told me that her workweek had just been cut from five days to four, and the second speech pathologist at the center who worked with adults had been laid off. The center seemed in a bit of a financial crisis, and Linda herself seemed besieged.

I asked her how typical I was. As it turned out, not typical at all. Many of her clients had hearing aids, and as they transitioned into cochlear implants, they would come back to her very soon after activation to continue audiotherapy. They were in a much better position to take advantage of the implant than someone like me, who started therapy six months after activation. She likes to begin working with an implant client the day after the implant is turned on. Audiotherapy generally takes about three months, and some clients come to her three times a week at the beginning.

I worked with Linda on auditory rehab rather than speechreading, but the therapy contained elements of both. "The more a client knows about the structure of a language and the sounds of a language," she told me, "the more they are able not just to hear words but to analyze sounds, the better they will be able to understand speech." Each therapy is individualized for the client, she said, but for most "to be able to say, for example, that one sound is a breath sound, another is a voice sound, enables them to listen better. It allows them to know how we speak and the nature of sound." Some people take to this method more quickly than others. "There are some people who come in here and grasp the theoretical information and there are some people whose brains just don't work that way. I think that's what happened to you."

Perhaps the biggest obstacle to success in my case, though, was the delay in starting therapy. This is not unusual. "Most audiologists believe that the implant will do its job eventually," she said. "It's when the client is having special problems that they'll refer them to a speech pathologist." The implant center in Ann Arbor, part of the University of Michigan Medical Center, is one of the few implant centers that build rehabilitative therapy into the implant process. That center, Linda told me, was started by a surgeon who said: "Therapy is vital following the implant. And no one will have an implant here without agreeing to and following through with therapy."

Linda is impatient with people who don't do their share of the therapy work. "If someone doesn't wear their implant," she said, "I say, 'Why are you coming? You don't wear it consistently. You don't practice.'" I heard that guiltily, thinking of the three months following my implant when I had done everything I could to ignore it.

Part of the problem for the center is that speech therapy is expensive and private insurance often doesn't cover it. Medicaid has just cut back its coverage for speech therapy, Linda told me. "In a whole calendar year, you now can only have twenty sessions of physical therapy, occupational therapy, and speech therapy combined, which means that if you have a stroke, you can forget it. This attitude toward therapy is ridiculous."

Linda also teaches group sessions in speechreading. My audiologist asked if I'd talk to a college instructor with hearing loss who was considering an implant. The first time we met, as we compared notes on our lives, I felt as if I'd met my doppelgänger. We were the same age, had lost our hearing at around the same time, both had a progressive loss, both got hearing aids at the same time from the same audiologist. We lived in the same neighborhood and she had even once lived in my building. She too had had fertility problems, but unlike me had taken that as an indication that she wasn't meant to have children. She was worried she might not be able to hear them, she told me. She was the first person I met who had gone through the same psychological reactions to hearing loss that I had. (Later I would meet many others.) We talked for quite a long time, our common backgrounds making us feel like old friends.

Another time when we met she told me that she took speechreading every week in a class with a dozen or so other adults. She said she'd found it very helpful and she liked the teacher very much. It turned out to be Linda Kessler.

Speechreading even for the very practiced is difficult. The journalist Henry Kisor, deaf since the age of three, relied entirely on speechreading. The title of his memoir of deafness, *What's That Pig Outdoors?*, illustrates the pitfalls of speechreading. Suffering from the flu, he writes, "suddenly and prodigiously I broke wind. My elder son, Colin, then five years old, dashed in wide-eyed from the kitchen and inquired, 'What's that big loud noise?' Mystified, I arose from the couch, peered out the window, and said 'What pig outdoors?'" His son stared at him, dumbfounded. "Go ahead," Kisor tells the reader, "look in the mirror and watch your lips: to a lip-reader 'What's that big loud noise?' looks exactly like 'What's that pig outdoors?'"

Kisor wrote that the secret to speechreading is "'context guessing,' the ability to fill in the gaps between words that are understood." As he points out, the letters *m, p,* and *b* all look alike on the lips, as do *t, d, n,* and *l*. As anyone who has taken aural rehabilitation or speechreading courses knows, the words "bat," "bad," "ban," "mat," "mad," "man," "pat," "pad," "pan" all look exactly alike on the lips. Combine that with low-frequency hearing loss, where the vowel sounds fall, and they all sound alike too. Once again, context is everything.

• • •

In July I started aural rehabilitation again, this time with Elizabeth Ying at the Cochlear Implant Center at the Ear Institute (part of the New York Eye and Ear Infirmary), where I got my implant. Liz was the director of what at NYEE is called Hearing Habilitation. What we practiced here, true to its name, was *hearing* rather than speech, which was what Linda Kessler seemed more focused on.

Liz usually works with children and she was interested to see what working with an adult would be like, so after my initial screening she took me on herself rather than delegating me to one of the other specialists in her department. Every Wednesday from four to five, we sat at a round table in her office surrounded by toys and colorful posters and a bulletin board covered with photographs of the children she's helped. Liz is sunny, with warm brown skin and, in the summertime, freckles across her nose, and her smile and ready laugh were reassuring and inviting. If I resented Linda (even as I recognized her skill and goodwill), I wanted to do my very best for Liz.

Tour, four, shore, chore. Fish, fist, fifth, fit. A hearing person might have a hard time understanding why these are so difficult to distinguish. Sheet/shoot. Pig/big. Park/bark. Cheap/jeep. Zoo/chew.

Each therapy session began with sounds. Liz would cover her mouth with the round crochet frame that all the speech therapists seem to use (to prevent lipreading) and ask me to repeat after her, one sound at a time: ah, ee, oo, mmm, ssss, sh. When I got one right, she'd triumphantly show me a card with the sound printed on it and a picture. "Ee" was illustrated with a bee, "oo" with a cow (moo), "s" with a snake. For months I continued to confuse "mmm" with "ee." I could always get "s" and "sh."

Liz and the hearing habilitation team at NYEE use what she described as an auditory-based approach, as opposed to a visually based program. "You can do visually based auditory training using the same kinds of materials"—words, sounds, sentences—with more of a focus on lipreading. Both Linda and Liz used the crochet hoop to keep me from seeing their lips as they talked, but Linda also included speechreading and teaching the mechanics of sound in her program.

I was one of just twelve adult clients a year at NYEE. Auditory rehab, as Linda said, is not considered important for adults, who it is assumed will naturally regain their hearing as they use the implant and do exercises provided online. There isn't a lot of funding for speech pathology, except with children, where it is mandated—at least in New York State. Most rehab classes are taught by audiologists rather than speech pathologists. "It's really a case of lack of funding and interest," Liz said. They simply can't find enough adequately trained speech pathologists to keep up with demand.

Private insurance will sometimes pay for rehabilitation if it is with a speech pathologist. My insurance reimbursed my sessions with Liz, but only up to twelve per calendar year. Adult post-implant therapy is by necessity highly individualized. "We may be working with a flight attendant who wants to get back to flying," Liz said, "or a social worker who needs to be able to make phone calls. For that person I'm really focusing on name recognition, a lot of phone practice." Liz and her colleagues take a pragmatic approach: "Some people just need to know how to get along at the grocery store." Each of the four clinicians at the implant center takes one adult for the twelve-week course, in addition to the children they're working with. The general practice is for the client to come back the following year, once their needs have become clearer, and focus more narrowly during the second twelve-week session.

Liz and I always had a conversation as part of our session. What we did over the weekend, perhaps, or what we had for dinner the evening before. I learned that she was about my age and had a daughter. At one point in the twelve-week course we were both dealing with sick elderly relatives, and we talked about that. Liz missed her sixtieth-birthday trip to the Caribbean because a favorite aunt had died, and we talked about that. My father died shortly after, and we talked about that.

Other times we'd practice everyday exchanges. How are you? What's your name? Hard, believe me. Then she would read—and reread—a passage and I'd try to summarize it. I couldn't get it at all the first time around, and sometimes not even the second or third. Sometimes she'd give me a hint. It's about business, she'd say. Then she'd read it again and I'd begin to distinguish words. Silicon Valley. Initial public offering. Once I began to get some words, the others would come more easily. In the end, I usually got about three-quarters of the words.

To my surprise and disappointment (and Liz's, I think), when I started my second twelve-week course I had fallen back almost to where I was when I started the first session. I could not tell the difference between "ee" and "mm"—they sounded identical, though they don't sound identical when I say them to myself. It is at least partly my fault. I am not a good patient. I don't work hard enough, I am distracted by almost every other element in my life. Everything comes before hearing practice: writing, working, reading, visiting my elderly mother, exercising, cooking, shopping, going to doctors, driving to the country, seeing friends and family.

I've been coasting on my facility with language, which did actually get me pretty far. "Being a writer, being in a field that is so linguistically based, so lexically based," Liz said, "you have the ability to fill in gaps with your skills that someone else might not have. I had a bus driver who had driven a bus for fifty years. He didn't fill in like that, it wasn't an automatic thing."

When I asked why they were able to take so few adults for auditory rehab, I heard a refrain that I'd heard already from Linda Kessler. "Here at the hospital they won't give me the staff," Liz said with evident frustration. "We don't have the fiscal support, the resources that would allow me to do this. Otherwise I would gladly opt for this as a routine thing. Medicare does not reimburse anything for therapy. Medicaid, I think it's about six dollars per session. So you've got to have good private insurance. A lot of private insurances don't do it, they don't see the benefit, they've already spent

$70,000 [for the implant] on you. So I know the cost of providing the service really limits a lot of agencies from doing it." There's another deterrent as well: "the expertise of the people doing it—they would rather work with the kids than with the adults. They don't know what to do with the adults."

• • •

In the fall of 2011, I visited Geoff Plant at the Hearing Rehabilitation Foundation in Somerville, Massachusetts. If Linda Kessler and Liz Ying feel the financial crunch, they should meet Geoff Plant. (Actually, both of them do know him: the world of auditory rehab is a small one.) The Hearing Rehabilitation Foundation occupies the second floor of a nondescript office building in a run-down area of Somerville, a suburb of Boston. My aunt, a lifelong resident of Somerville and now Cambridge, offered to drive me there but then had no idea how to find it. We had to call Plant several times along the way for updated directions.

Geoff Plant is an expansive talker with wide-ranging interests. He was wearing jeans and a sweatshirt, sneakers. He apologized for the frigid temperature in the room: they can't afford the heat. Geoff *is* the Hearing Rehabilitation Foundation to a large extent, though he works there only on Fridays and Saturdays and on a volunteer basis. The other four days of the week he is a consultant to MED-EL U.K., through their office in England. The work he does at the Rehabilitation Foundation is clearly a labor of love and intellectual curiosity. His enthusiasm is contagious, and those he works with—from well-known musicians to neighborhood schoolchildren—seem devoted to him. When I talked to Ben Luxon, the one person he urged me to meet was Geoff Plant.

His "desk" was piled high with electronic components, and several computer screens sat close by—all part of his work. Around the edges of the big cold room were piles and piles of boxes, a sagging couch, and a small musical instrument that I later learned was a baritone ukulele, which he uses in his therapy. Plant charges a meager sum to those he works with, and has no pretensions to elegant furnishings or an expensive neighborhood. He'd rather spend the money helping people hear again.

I asked Plant how he and Ben Luxon had met. The answer was characteristically digressive—a story that unfolded as it went on. "Do you know, I can't remember how we got to meet each other," he began in his Australian accent. "We [no hint as to who "we" were] were living in Sweden about eighteen years ago, and someone had come to Boston and had got an article out of *The Boston Globe* about this opera singer who was going deaf. It was a terrible story because Richard Dyer, who was the music critic at that time for the *Globe*, had written a scathing review of Ben's performance, without realizing what had happened.

"I remember reading the article and thinking how interesting it was, and I actually brought it with me when we moved to the United States. I was up in my office, cleaning up my office, and I came across this newspaper article, which I had brought with me, and I read it again, and thought, 'Oh, that's interesting,' and about an hour later Susie [Susie Crofut, Ben's wife] rang me, and it was really, really strange. She was describing her husband and all of these problems, and I finally said, 'Is his name Ben Luxon?'" It was, of course.

"At that time there wasn't a lot I could do for Ben, because his communication skills were relatively good, he wasn't really a cochlear implant candidate, and I'll have to admit I wasn't all that keen on him getting one anyway, because of his music. What he wanted his hearing for was for music, and I wasn't confident that that was going to be a great success. So we saw each other on and off for quite a while, and then again we lost contact."

Ben did get an implant, and several years later got back in touch with Geoff. "His listening skills were pretty impressive, but they're far more impressive now; he's really, he's very good, but music is still a problem, as I'm sure he's told you. I found myself in this very strange situation, the last time I saw him, which was . . . I asked him because of a story he had told me, actually that Susie had told me . . . I asked him to sing 'Simple Gifts' for me, and he sang it in his full-blown operatic voice and it wasn't great . . . and I was a little taken aback by the fact that it just wasn't good at all, and wasn't holding the tune very well, so I asked him to sing it again, but this time sing it like I did, and I sang it as [sings in a talking voice] ''Tis the gift to be simple, 'tis the gift to be free . . .' Very much a non-trained voice, and he sang it and it sounded so much better."

Ben couldn't hear his voice when he sang operatically. He had no idea whether he was on pitch or not. But using a kind of Rex Harrison song/speaking voice, he could hear himself.

Working with Ben, Geoff said, "confirmed a belief I've had for a long time that trained voices are probably not good voices for implant listening, there's too much going on." A trained opera singer, who must project his voice over an orchestra, develops modifications to his vocal tract, something called "the singer's formant," which, Geoff said, "produces a big heap of sound at a place where you wouldn't normally find it." Trained opera singers, especially men, have a formant, or peak sound, at about 3000 hz, which is not true in the untrained voice. The singer's formant allows the un-amplified voice to be heard over the orchestra. Because an implant is designed for a speaking voice, when Ben was singing in his oper-atic voice he could not hear himself, he couldn't hear the pitch. But when he sang in a more conversational, untrained way, he could.

The same holds true for an implant user who is not a trained musician. It is usually much more difficult to listen to opera, because the implant processor cannot deal with the pitch in the singer's formant, Geoff said. He played a video of Johnny Cash singing "I Walk the Line": "I keep a close watch on this heart of mine/I keep my eyes wide open all the time/I keep the ends out for the tie that binds/Because you're mine, I walk the line . . ."

"How does it sound?" he asked. It sounded fine, I told him. I could hear the tone of Cash's voice, and because it was subtitled I could understand the words. He tells his clients to listen to music this way and soon they will become better and better at hearing music. You go onto YouTube, "you type in what you want to hear, and add the word 'lyrics,' you can do things like this . . ." He plays "Yesterday" by the Beatles. It sounds terrible. "Are they playing it the way it was originally recorded?" I asked. Geoff said they might have reedited and remixed it, or maybe Paul McCartney's voice is at a frequency level that I don't have access to anymore.

Geoff Plant trained as a teacher of the deaf but identifies most closely with hearing therapists. He is one of the few therapists who use music in their training, with musicians and nonmusicians. He had worked with Richard Reed, whom I heard talk and play at the HLAA conference in 2011. Reed did not mention Plant by name but told the audience he had gone to a speech therapist after getting his implant. He "got" speech so quickly that the therapist had suggested they work on music.

Reed described his first days with the implant with entertaining and quite funny staccato showmanship: "I started the car," he said. "VROOM. The radio was noise, high-pitched, like cartoon weasels arguing.

"From the sounds of silence I went to hearing percussive noises everywhere," he went on. "The sound of walking, my corduroys rubbing. Family and friends sounded like giant chipmunks, but I could understand them. The next morning I had the noisiest breakfast. The cereal flakes falling in the bowl, the clank of the spoon. I went down to the beach. It was as if the sky was filled with wind chimes. I realized it was the foam coming to shore. Those high pitches, my brain turned them into little bells."

Geoff Plant invited me to watch him working with a client. He uses pitch and rhythm even when he's not using music. While we waited for the client, he explained: "I use mainly connected speech. So I do a lot of work in sentences; paragraphs, even. There are two kinds of approaches—one is called 'analytic' and the other 'synthetic'—and I don't actually believe in either of them; I believe that you've got to do the two of them together. So I try to have some aspects of the analytic, which is 'Did I say "bib" or "Bob,"' that sort of stuff; that's the analytic training . . ."

"I didn't hear the two words you said," I said. "Did you say, 'I say what or what'?"

"Bib" or "Bob."

Me: "Bim" or "Bomb"? Did I get that right?

No, Bib.

Me: "B-I-M?"

No, B-I-B.

Me, finally: "Ah, or Bob . . ."

The client was a teenage boy with a multitude of problems and an endearing determination to learn. His mother drives him into Somerville after school gets out. He has an implant and a hearing aid. After a few preliminaries, he sat down across the desk from Geoff. His name was Oberon.

Geoff began in a fast rhythmic pace: "Okay, are you ready, let's do that thing we do, 'Oberon, Oberon, Oberon,' can you do that . . . 'Oberon, Oberon, Oberon, and Geoff . . . My name is Oberon, your name is Geoff . . . Oberon, Oberon, Oberon, and Geoff,' now you do it . . ."

Oberon repeated it, somewhat haltingly.

Geoff: "That's fantastic, you sound so good, are you ready to do this one? Here we go: 'Five, four, three, two, one!'" Oberon repeated it, and then Geoff did it again, back and forth, until finally Oberon stumbled halfway through. "Whoops, start again," Geoff said, making a fake snoring sound. "I'm going to go to sleep, I'm afraid, c'mon! Let's do it together: 'Five, four, three, two, one, you and I have lots of fun. Five, four, three, two, one, in the snow, and in the sun. Five, four, three, two, one, when we walk, and when we run. Five, four, three, two, one, you and I have lots of fun.' Now you do it that way, come on . . . and if I go to sleep, you'll know it's wrong." Oberon gamely started out, then tripped up halfway through on "in the snow." "Oh! Too slow!" Geoff said. "C'mon . . . [Oberon completed the rest] . . . That was pretty good, I like that anyway . . ."

Then Geoff moved on to another exercise, just as rapid-fire:

"Ready," he said. "What color is that? What about this one?

What's that one? . . . That one? That one? That one?" As Geoff flipped the color cards, Oberon named them.

"Okay, well done, you're doing really well. You ready? Here we go, show me yellow, too slow, yellow. Show me gray. Show me black, show me pink, show me red, show me orange. Now two: show me white and yellow, show me purple and black, show me orange and red [Oberon: "Say again, please?"], orange and red. ["Orange and gray."] Nope! Orange and red. Piece of cake for you! So good!"

Oberon's mother's cell phone rang. "Your mother's phone makes a cool noise, okay, are you ready? Oberon is quite shy today, isn't he? This is funny." And he started in again on another repetitive rhythmic series of words, which Oberon repeated: "Pineapple, pineapple, I love pineapple! Pineapple, pineapple . . . Pineapple, pineapple on my plate! Pineapple, pineapple, it tastes great!"

Geoff and Oberon will go for more than an hour. I was exhilarated, exhausted, freezing, and both relieved and sorry when my aunt called up to say she was out front.

Geoff invited me to come up and work with him for an afternoon. After watching him with Oberon, I don't think I have the stamina for it. The work is fast-paced, totally different from that of any of the speech therapists I've seen, clearly fun as well as very hard work on the part of the client. And if Oberon, Ben, and Richard Reed are examples, it's an intriguingly successful technique.

VOICES: KARIN OLSOE

Nursing, like most jobs in medicine, would seem to require good hearing. Karin Olsoe began to lose hers when she was already well into her nursing career. After six or seven years of progressively worsening hearing, she said, "I no longer could hear the IV pump alarms or a patient's call button." She relied on her memory to prompt her to change an IV.

"Working with patients, I would often need them to repeat what they said." In the postoperative room, there might be four patients in addition to families and friends, creating overlapping noise that made it difficult to get information that she needed. She would be "literally in their face" to get crucial information. When it came to insignificant information, she faked it: "I would pretend I heard them, nod, laugh . . ."

Several times, physicians would become irritated when she didn't understand their orders correctly. She would be, as she said, "holding back tears, feeling stupid and inadequate." She relied on colleagues to take phone reports or orders for her, to ensure she got them right. She never told the physicians, since she saw them irregularly and some only occasionally. But her fellow nurses and others backed her up when necessary.

Karin is now studying for a master's in nursing. In an essay she wrote for a class on social injustice, she described herself as "privileged." Her parents were immigrants from Norway, and she grew up on the East Coast and in Norway. Her father, whose first job in New York was as a cake decorator at the Waldorf-Astoria, was a building contractor and became successful enough over the years to pay for his daughter to go to college, and even to buy her a car her senior year.

Karin lives in Seattle, near the University of Washington. She began to lose her hearing when she was thirty-five and pregnant with her third child. She noticed herself saying, "What did you say?" Her family noticed it too. Although her grandmother had significant hearing loss and tinnitus and one of her sisters had a mild hearing loss, she said, "it never occurred to me that there could be a genetic component." She got hearing aids, which she refused to wear. She lost the first pair within a month. With the second set, she finally adjusted to them, and acknowledged that she heard better with them. She had expected her hearing would "miraculously" come back to normal with the hearing aids. It didn't, of course.

Eventually, after too many passed-along phone calls and impatient doctors, she left the job. She heard too well to qualify for disability. She withdrew, avoided social situations, texted on her cell phone rather than talk, worked as a home health aide for a retired minister. Then, when she was fifty, she got a cochlear implant. The experience, she wrote, was "amazing." She could hear the rain, the turn signal in the car, the rustling of paper.

It took three years for her to be able to use the phone, and by then she was ready to go back to work. She took an RN refresher course, got a per diem job at her old hospital, and in July of 2011 got a second cochlear implant.

"So today I sit here and see how privileged I am!" she wrote in her essay. What if she were not from a middle-class family and without a college education and medical insurance. "Would I still be deaf?" she asked. With her hearing loss, she wrote, her status changed from someone privileged and unmarked to someone with a stigma. It made her more aware of the difficulties other people experience as part of everyday life. And it made her aware of how much she has to be thankful for.

TEN

How to Be a Deaf Theater Editor, and Other Challenges of Real Life

In the summer of 2008, after almost ten years as deputy editor at the *Times Magazine*, I was appointed books and theater editor on the daily paper. A challenge for anyone, but especially someone with faulty hearing. I explained my hearing situation to Sam Sifton, my new boss, before accepting the job. But I underestimated the difficulties and overestimated my ability to handle them: not only was there a grueling amount of work, but learning the names of the many members of the Culture department, learning a new computer system, a new daily routine, a new kind of assigning and editing—a new way of doing just about everything—rapidly took its toll.

From the time I started my job in the department, I knew I was in for a challenge. I oversaw all the daily and Sunday theater coverage, including reviews and features, as well as all the daily book reviews and features. I also edited the "Abroad" column written by Michael Kimmelman from Berlin. In the distant flush days of the *Times*, there was a daily books editor, a daily theater editor, a Sunday theater editor, and a Michael Kimmelman editor (the art editor, when Kimmelman was chief art critic). I figured I was doing the work of three and a half people. (Indeed, when I left the paper, at least one element was not taken over by my successor—editing Kimmelman, an elegant writer but a time-consuming perfectionist.) I had always worked on a Mac and had to adjust to a PC, as well as a daily and weekly routine that was full of deadlines. My own section was down two staff members (no third book critic and no theater reporter), so until the replacements were named I had to find freelancers to fill those assignments. My predecessor had left for a new job before I started. I was on my own for the most part, to sink or swim.

I managed to swim (flailing, head barely above water) until November of that year, three months after I started the job. At that point, I had my Halloween breakdown—it was a hearing breakdown but it felt like an emotional one as well. I never did recover my hearing. I had been having trouble hearing anyway, but now I panicked. I remember leading a meeting in November or early December with eight or ten people present, sitting around a small conference table. A few months earlier, I'd have been able to hear them. Now I couldn't. But I didn't tell anyone. Deftly (or so I thought), I asked each participant to send me a summary of their suggestions after the meeting. I could crib from them for my report and no one would be the wiser (or so I thought).

People who lose their hearing are afraid to be open about it because they fear the reaction—the prejudice, fear of seeming old or stupid. But what really makes you seem old or stupid, I know now, is *not* acknowledging the handicap. You ask the wrong questions or give the wrong answers; you seem vacant, not paying attention, maybe drunk, maybe senile. You can't be a "team player," as the boss who finally gave me the shove put it.

I did tell my close colleagues. I don't think they really understood the extent of my loss, but at least they knew there was a problem and made an effort to accommodate it.

First thing every morning in the Culture department was a meeting of the senior editors and the rest of the staff. Among the senior editors were those who covered classical music, pop music, art and architecture, movies, TV, and video games. I covered books and theater. There were about as many top editors: Sifton, who was culture editor until August 2009; three deputies; the day editor; the Sunday editor. Web editors, photo editors, designers, production editors, the copy chief, and editors from the media desk. Except on holidays there were usually at least twenty of us, gathered informally in an open space near the picture desk, some people sitting at desks, some on them, most standing or leaning over the partition. It looked like a classic movie version of a newspaper office, but tidier.

The Times Building is designed on an open plan. The theme is transparency. It looks great. But it's terrible acoustically. It's exactly the kind of architecture John Carey at Johns Hopkins was lamenting when he said that architects and engineers have "no understanding of the tremendous degradation to communication that results from failure to minimize background noise." Our morning meeting took place near an atrium opening to the main news floor below. Even early in the morning, before the newsroom activity escalated, sound drifted up. Voices were swallowed by the space.

It was fifteen minutes of anxiety. And it was the start of every single morning. No matter where I stood or sat, someone on the other side of the room was too far away for me to hear. The one person I really needed to hear on any given day was invariably on the far side of the group. Or Sam would not be in his usual place, meaning that positioning myself near where he ordinarily stood did me no good. I couldn't hear anyone with a beard or mustache, because I couldn't read their lips. People talked very fast, or over each other, or very, very quietly.

Each subject editor would discuss the stories he or she had in progress, what kind of placement the story should get. Should it be pitched for Page One of the main paper? Did it break news, mine new territory, make a global point? Could it hold for another day if it didn't make Page One that day? For how long?

More often, the subject editor described the contents of a review or feature and where and when it should run. The "dress page"—the front page of the arts section—was premium real estate. Whether a story or a review was placed there depended on how important the subject was, how well written the piece was, how good the art accompanying it was, what the mix of the page was that day. It also depended on who was writing it: a glowing review by one of the chief critics trumped a glowing review by a second-tier critic, a feature by one of the favorite reporters was more likely to run on the section's front page than a feature by someone else. So was a story that one of the paper's top editors (Bill Keller or Jill Abramson) had suggested. Competition for the space was fierce. Everything else went inside the arts section—often, it felt, never to be read. Especially on a Saturday. Reporters would beg me to keep their features out of the Saturday paper.

If an editor had a breaking news story, there might be a discussion about how the reporting was going and what time the story would be filed. It was important not only to hear the questions, but also the answers. I could usually get what was said directly to me, sometimes with help from whoever was nearby, but rarely could I hear what was said to (or by) my fellow editors. I'd wait until the daily schedule came around an hour later and figure it out by working backward. I never could hear well enough to know what the discussion was, so I rarely said anything.

I spent many hours with Therese, my audiologist, and with my psychotherapist, rejecting their suggestions for how I could hear better in these meetings. Each solution would have meant involving other people in my deafness. Therese suggested a device I could put on the desk to receive signals and transmit them to my hearing aid. But that meant that each of the other speakers had to have a small mike. One of her patients, a CEO, used it for board meetings. I pointed out that I was a lot lower on the totem pole. So I stumbled and faltered and misheard and misspoke.

I didn't get the implant until almost a year later, a year with no hearing in one ear and very impaired hearing in the other. Even after I got the implant, I struggled.

It would have been hard enough in any job, but as theater editor I went to the theater two or three times a week. I couldn't hear with the infrared hearing devices many theaters provide (which require you to take off your hearing aid), but I read the plays in advance and read the actors' lips. I probably would not have worn the headphones anyway. It didn't seem like a good idea to advertise that the *Times*'s theater editor couldn't hear. Theaters now sometimes have devices you wear around your neck that pick up dialogue from a transmitter and deliver it directly to your hearing aid or cochlear implant. It's more discreet than the infrared devices, and it works better. Theaters outside of New York are sometimes looped.

As the *Times*'s theater editor, I had the best seat in the house, sixth or seventh row aisle. Sometimes I felt like I was walking in on a red carpet. Despite the great seat, close enough to read the actors' lips, I still missed way too much. But not so much that I couldn't assign stories on actors and composers and costume designers, on theatrical legends making one last star turn, on an interesting new playwright or actor.

I couldn't tolerate Broadway musicals, however, which are invariably overamplified. I remember seeing *Billy Elliot*, probably on opening night, sitting in the sixth or seventh row, the orchestra pit just twenty feet in front of me. I loved the show but the music was an enveloping cacophony, discordant, dissonant, deafening (even for someone who was already deaf). My sister, who had gone with me and has perfect hearing, had her fingers in her ears for the whole two hours and forty-five minutes. At *Next to Normal*, about a mother's bipolar disorder, I was the only dry-eyed person in the audience, because I had no idea what the words to the songs were. But I saw every major Broadway and Off-Broadway show in the 2008–2009 theater season. And it was a great season, one of the best in years.

As books editor, the other half of my job, I met frequently with editors and publicists who wanted to discuss their lists. I tried always to meet them in a small, acoustically favorable room, but some voices were impossible to hear, some accents made comprehension difficult, noise in the hall drowned out noise in the closed conference room. I was also sometimes invited to small fancy lunches to introduce new books. A publisher would invite ten or twenty editors and writers and influential bookstore owners to lunch at Gramercy Tavern or the Modern (at the Museum of Modern Art), once even at Le Bernardin. The food was always delicious and when the writer spoke I could sometimes hear what he or she said about the new book. But I could never hear the table conversation before the formal presentation. I stopped going to those lunches because they made me too uncomfortable. I felt, as I often did, stupid.

I communicated with my writers as much as possible either face-to-face, where I could read their lips, or by e-mail. I e-mailed people who were ten feet away. But there were a couple of writers who wanted to talk—by phone. Often those calls would go on for a half hour or forty minutes, with me catching just as much as I needed to murmur occasionally, "That sounds good," "Oh, I'm so sorry," or "Well, just get it to me as soon as you can."

I couldn't hear the office banter, and although I had smart and amusing neighbors—Chip McGrath and David Carr among them—I couldn't join in the conversation. I missed gossip, I missed jokes, I missed announcements, I missed arguments, I missed the occasional dressing-down of someone or praise lavished by a senior editor. I pretended to laugh or to look shocked or to nod sagely when it seemed appropriate. But again, I never knew whether my response was indeed appropriate or somehow completely off the mark.

Once or twice, Sam Sifton asked if I would go to the Page One meeting, where the masthead editors decide what will go on the front page of the next day's paper. You represent your department at the meeting, attended by department heads and senior editors as well as the managing editor, then Jill Abramson, and the executive editor, then Bill Keller. The meeting had grown since I first started attending it as deputy science editor in the late nineties. Max Frankel, executive editor, sat at one end of a much smaller table, with

Joe Lelyveld at the other. Max Frankel especially would question you closely about your story, often spotting the holes or inconsistencies in your summary. It was hard, but I enjoyed it.

When I was in Culture, I was not a regular at the meeting and never got the rhythm. I would make a case for Page One worthiness for the story I was representing—and then the questions came from Bill or Jill, a football field away, down at the other end of the table. True panic was seeing Jill raise her eyebrows and direct a question to me that I couldn't begin to hear.

I heard just as badly with the implant for the first few months. It was a relief to know that I could hear *something* with the implant, that I would never be deaf. But it wasn't enough to help me at work. I now know that this is not an unusual experience. It can take up to two years for an adult to get the full benefit of the implant, and that full benefit may then still be relatively meager. One point of the psychological workup before you're implanted is to ensure that your expectations are not too high. It also helps if the expectations of those around you are not too high. My expectations were reasonable: I hoped to be able to function better in my job. I didn't expect to be able to hear as I once had. I just wanted to comprehend speech. But even this expectation couldn't be met.

I managed with the backing of an understanding boss and colleagues. The hearing setbacks were frustrating but not prohibitive. It was only when a new culture editor came into the department that I faltered. Without his confidence, I lost mine, and I could no longer do the job. It was this editor who told me I wasn't a "team player" and said I wasn't "on board" with the program. I've always hated this kind of corporate-speak and bristled at the language. I was also deeply sad to realize that my time in the job was at an end.

I was protected under the Americans with Disabilities Act, which defines as a disability a physical or mental condition that substantially limits a major life activity (such as walking, talking, seeing, hearing, or learning). The act forbids discrimination in any aspect of employment: hiring, firing, pay, job assignments, promotions, layoff, training, fringe benefits, etc. But—and this was a big *but* for me and is for many people with hearing loss—in order to be protected under the act, I had to acknowledge my disability. I had to ask for accommodations that would have permitted me to do my job. The ball was in my court, and I refused to play. Rather than acknowledge my disability, I walked out.

In the spring of 2011, two New York City police officers filed a complaint with the Federal Equal Employment Opportunity Commission, after they were forced to retire on disability at ages forty-four and forty. Candidates for the police force now must pass a hearing test, but the Police Department used to allow officers to wear hearing aids on the job as long as they weren't visible. Thomas Graham, a former deputy chief, wore a hearing aid, and he said he knew of no policy forbidding them during his thirty-seven years on the force. "If you wanted a hearing aid, as long as it's not pink and dangling out of your ear, nobody is going to bother you over it," said Mr. Graham, who had retired the year before, at age sixty-three.

The police department had paid $3000 for a hearing aid for one of the involuntarily retired officers just months before he was put on disability. A police department spokesman, Paul J. Browne, was quoted by the *Times* as saying that hearing aids were "incompatible with police work because they were vulnerable to mechanical failure, earwax buildup or any number of things," and could not "completely compensate for hearing deficiencies that might render an officer unable to hear a command properly."

This caused an uproar in the disability rights community, but as someone with hearing aids (as well as a cochlear implant), I have to agree with the policy. My hearing aid battery is always going dead when I don't expect it to. The battery beeps a warning before it dies, and I carry spares, but it takes time to change the battery. As for the implant, the battery goes dead without warning. And as I've said, it can be brushed off or knocked off fairly easily. I don't want someone like me pulling a gun on criminals, responding to fires, working for the EMS, flying a plane, or doing any of a variety of other jobs where hearing well is crucial. Following my own dictum, I no longer sit in the emergency exit rows on airplanes, and although I used to be certified in CPR, I have let my certification lapse. There are some times and places where hearing is nonnegotiable. The police commissioner, Raymond W. Kelly, by the way, wears hearing aids in both ears, but as a civilian he is exempt from both age and physical requirements.

I admire those police officers. I was too ashamed of my hearing loss, fearful that people would misinterpret it as a sign of aging or weakness, unfitness for the competitive world of the newspaper (where I had, after all, managed to compete quite successfully for twenty-two years). I let my new boss accuse me of not being a team player, of not fitting into the department, rather than explain to him why I was the way I was. Even when I appealed his decision to the assistant managing editor who was *his* boss, I never mentioned my deafness.

Why was this? And why *is* this the situation for so many hearing-impaired people? Hearing loss is a hidden disability. We can pretend it doesn't exist. I feared that once my hearing loss was known, I would be identified first and always as a person with hearing loss, and only second and incidentally as a skilled editor and writer, a good manager, a disciplined and organized supervisor able to bring those traits out in others. I didn't want my disability to define me.

· · ·

E-mail is the best thing that's ever happened for the hard of hearing, even for people who can't or don't want to type an e-mail. I've gotten e-mails written using voice-activated software that came through without a glitch.

E-mail was how I got through the last year at the *Times* when I was so deaf. I could barely hear on the phone (and was grateful for caller ID). If someone called, or if I didn't quite get what was said in person, I'd say casually, "Can you follow up with an e-mail? I'm really distracted right now." If the caller ID didn't identify the caller, I might not know to whom I was talking until I got the follow-up e-mail.

I used e-mail in my personal life too, training friends and family (all except my mother) to communicate in writing. Instant messaging, texting, G-chat, Skype, Facebook, Twitter, Tumblr (whatever that is) are all preferred means of communicating for busy youth, so you can feel hip rather than impaired using them.

• • •

Even with my implant and my hearing aid and my devices and the best doctors and resources, I still don't hear many things that may seem trivial until you no longer can hear them.

I can no longer hear a whisper, but I remember the feel of it: warm breath in your ear, the intimacy of a mouth close enough almost to touch, the pleasure of words meant just for you. And the response: the secret smile of acknowledgment, the burst of laughter, the gasp of astonishment or horror.

I remember overheard conversations, in a restaurant, on a train, snippets of a life that could be spun into a story if you were so inclined.

I remember the sound of someone calling my name from across a street, a wave, a chance meeting with an old friend.

I remember the discomfort at hearing muttered words of anger or jokes at someone's expense, words the speaker would immediately like to retract. And I remember the power it gives you to have heard them—to withhold and protect the speaker, or to use them.

As I was writing this, the term "Shouts and Murmurs" kept running through my head, like a refrain, probably because I don't hear them either. *The New Yorker* uses the rubric "Shouts & Murmurs" for its humor column. Murmurs are not quite whispers; in fact, in some ways they are the opposite: comments made in an offhand way that suggests the speaker is not really sure he (or she) wants to be heard. Murmurs can also be the low, steady noise of a crowd, or a swarm of bees, or a whoosh in the heart that shouldn't be there.

As for shouts, from another room they sound like barks, or a loud male sneeze, or a door slamming. My husband sneezes and I yell "What?" and he shouts back something that could be anything. Irritated, I tromp into the room. "What?" I say. "Nothing," he says, "I just sneezed.'"

In conversation, when people think I haven't heard them, they may lean in close and shout. I jump back. Even my $3000 hearing aid lacks that effective tempering mechanism—nowhere as good as the human ear's—that allows the ear to adjust to a noise. And if I can't see the person, if I can't read their lips, I can't hear them. So it's a double negative—too loud, and too little available information.

• • •

The great unspoken fact about hearing aids and implants is that even the best hearing devices often are not enough. It's no wonder that the audiologist or superstore or website selling you that $2000-to-$6000 hearing aid may be reluctant to mention that you may need to shell out another few thousand to really get the full benefit. But these devices might have helped me and others.

In 2011, I attended a conference at Gallaudet to train people about the kinds of assistive technologies that are available to supplement hearing aids and cochlear implants. I already had some of them: The iCom Bluetooth device that transmitted sound from my cell phone (or iPod or laptop) directly into my hearing aid. An amplified telephone. My Sun Rise Alarm clock that mimics dawn shining into my dark bedroom. Access to a captioned calling system.

Since I am fairly deaf in my "good" ear, even with my hearing aid, I still don't hear well on the phone. So when I am at my desk I use a captioned relay system, which is provided free to people with hearing loss. The one I use is ClearCaptions.com. To make a call I go on my computer, sign on to ClearCaptions, type in the number I'm calling to and the number I'm calling from. A few seconds later, my desk phone rings and I get a notice on my laptop screen that I am now connected to Captioner 147845 or some other string of numbers. I hear the phone at the other end ring. When it is picked up, the Captioner (I'm not sure if it's a human or a voice-activated computer) begins typing. The person I call most often on the phone is my mother, who lives at the Preston Health Center. (She is unable to e-mail or use Skype, or even really to fully follow a conversation.)

At the Preston, the person answering the phone says, "Good afternoon. Preston Health Center. This is Laura [or whoever is answering] speaking. How may I help you?"

ClearCaptions hears this as, variously:

"Good afternoon, A Person healthcare. Is the Lord speaking."

"Good Morning, Oppressive Health Care."

"Good Morning, Apprentice Health Care. Dolor speaking."

"Good Morning, Custom Health Center."

Another call, to WageWorks:

"Good morning, Weight Works."

I ask my question.

"Mably chewable wad do some research for you," the captions say.

I translate this as "May I put you on hold while I do some research for you."

To Vanguard (it happens to be Valentine's Day):

"Thank you for calling Vanguard Flagship Services.

"You have reached avoids launches the lonely this Tuesday, February 14. I am at the office today but with my desk Romulan woman.

"If this call records immediate assistance, please press 0 to speak to another colleague at the flagship."

I could switch captioning systems and probably get one that would be more accurate. But this one is too much fun.

The network news broadcasts are all captioned. They make even the dreariest news amusing, with phrases like these, the intention of most of which I couldn't figure out:

The boy ate the bridge
Can you hear the garbage
He liked to eat morphine
Argue nick (Ah, I think, that one must be "arsenic.")
Totaled 15 winds over all
I'm gonna bring my sleeping back
Stripped of his medical lie sense
Knelt unyahu (Netanyahu)
For a selth straight day (Seventh? Twelfth? Somewhere in
     between?)
Blahmahsan Boar Genie (which had something to do with
     a Lamborghini)
Sharing this trautic story (traumatic). Oh dear.

• • •

There was much discussion at the Gallaudet meeting about hearing loops, which are regarded by some as almost as miraculous as the hearing aid. I came away from the three-day conference thinking that maybe I would be able to hear again—in a group, in a restaurant, in a meeting. It all sounded so promising and so easy. But when it came to an FM system for myself, with a cochlear implant in one ear and a hearing aid (and severe hearing loss) in the other, I was lost. It was a few months after this meeting that Therese and I embarked on the four months of fitting and refitting, of finding that what worked with the hearing aid did not work with the cochlear implant.

Eventually Therese and Megan and I decided that Megan should handle both my cochlear implant and my hearing aid. It was just too difficult to coordinate between two audiologists. Megan ordered me yet another new hearing aid, and this one worked well right from the start. Both cochlear implant and hearing aid had telecoils. I already owned the MyLink/SmartLink system, which worked with both. Theoretically, I was set!

Theoretically. In practice, I couldn't program the MyLink/

SmartLink to work with my iPhone, so I continued to use the iCom. In practice, I found the FM system less than perfect. In groups like my book club, the MyLink/SmartLink involved either passing the transmitter around from one person to another to speak into directly or setting it on the table, where it picked up a lot of background noise. As mentioned earlier, people in groups—and especially my lively book club—tend to speak over one another.

But in the spring of 2012, the FM system opened up a whole new opportunity for me. I've always loved to travel, but I no longer had the courage—without my hearing—to travel alone. I signed up for a tour of China sponsored by my college, following the Silk Road to Kashgar, close to the western border of China and bordering Kyrgystan. There were eight of us on the tour—all women, as it happened. The guide wore my FM transmitter and I wore the receiver. It was a triumphant success. There was another hearing-impaired woman on the trip—not as bad off as me—but thanks to the FM system, I was able to fill her in on a few missed details. That is, for me, a rare experience.

• • •

Just after that trip I heard looping for the first time—in June of 2012, at the 2012 HLAA annual conference. I set both hearing aid and cochlear implant to the telecoil mode, and I heard as well as I had heard in many, many years. It was, as promised, nothing short of miraculous. But it was, so far, an isolated event. I had not before then and have not since encountered a looped environment. John Tierney's 2011 *New York Times* article had mentioned a number of places in New York City where looping could be found. Among those he mentioned were the ticket windows of New York's two baseball stadiums, Yankee Stadium and Citi Field. Ellis Island is looped (I assume this means the information booth), as is the American Museum of Natural History and the Metropolitan Museum. So is the SoHo Apple store. The article went on: "Even in that infamous black hole of acoustics—the New York City subway system—loops are being placed in about 500 fare booths, in what will be the largest installation in the United States." I'm not sure what fare booths Tierney was referring to. In most if not all of the subway stations that I use, fare booths have been closed, replaced by machines. Some have even been removed.

For me, assistive technology is still a work in progress.

VOICES: ISAIAH JACKSON

Isaiah Jackson had a twenty-year career as a distinguished guest conductor with major orchestras around the world. Home base was Rochester, New York, where he was an associate conductor at the Rochester Philharmonic. He met his wife there and they raised three children. In 1987, he and his family moved to England, where he became principal conductor, then music director of the Royal Ballet at Covent Garden, a position he held until 1990.

He developed moderate to severe hearing loss in his right ear in 1995. Then, in 2004, he suffered sudden hearing loss in his left ear. It didn't stop him. He conducted wearing hearing aids. Orchestras, he said to me, can be predictable. "The things that happened they still happened. Pizzicato, where they rushed before, they still rushed." He used his eyes, he said: "If the concertmaster is at the tip of the bow, then all the strings need to be at the tip." He could fix style, he said, he could fix ensemble, he could see who played first. As for pitch, however, "that was a disaster." A common problem for those with hearing loss. "Everything above the A above middle C shifted up. It sounded terrible."

He stopped conducting, not because he couldn't do it but because he got no pleasure from the distortion in the sound. "I couldn't enjoy the music," he said. "In 2006 I said, 'Enough. I need to do something else. There's no point in doing things you don't enjoy.'" He was sixty-one.

Jackson went into music against his parents' wishes. He had started piano at age four, as therapy for a childhood injury. (He fell on a milk bottle and severed the tendons in his wrist.) By the time he was old enough for college, his father, an orthopedic surgeon in Richmond, Virginia, said he could major in anything but music. Jackson is black, and there were very few black classical musicians in the sixties when he went to college. At Harvard he dutifully majored in Russian history and literature, but he didn't give up music.

He joined the Harvard University choir and then aimed his ambitions at the Bach Society Orchestra, which was conducted by an undergraduate. First he needed to get some experience, however, so he and a group of friends decided to put on an opera: *Cosi fan Tutte* by Mozart. "Not a simple thing to start with," he said with a smile. "We had no business doing it." They recruited an orchestra and singers. The performance took place in Leverett House in the dining hall, also a Harvard tradition.

By then, other black classical musicians, like Henry Lewis (who later made his Metropolitan Opera debut in 1972), had begun to pave the way. From Harvard, Jackson went on to Stanford, getting an M.A. in music. He then studied with Nadia Boulanger in France before going to Juilliard, where he got a D.M.A. in conducting in 1973.

Like many musicians, Isaiah Jackson began to experience noise-related hearing loss; in his case, it was high-frequency loss in one ear from the flutes and piccolos rehearsing in a practice room. In 1995, though, he experienced a much more severe loss: sudden sensorineural hearing loss in his right ear. He was making coffee and out of nowhere his ear started ringing; when the ringing stopped, he couldn't hear. Though he was given immediate steroid treatment, the hearing did not come back. He still had fairly good hearing in his left ear, where the noise damage was, but high-frequency loss in both ears.

He continued to conduct, despite the deaf ear. "The halls are so acoustically good, you can hear everything. If I needed to hear the other side of the orchestra, I would turn. I didn't talk about it. I learned to fake it."

Then, in 2004, he suffered sudden hearing loss in his other ear, the left. Whatever pleasure he got from hearing the music he helped to make was gone.

Now he teaches at Berklee College of Music, where conducting is a required course. Berklee has a strong classical department, and teaching those students to conduct is relatively easy. But Berklee was founded as a jazz school and students majoring in jazz, Appalachian music, Latin music, or Indian music are harder to teach, since conducting is taught primarily with classical music.

Jackson, a meticulously soft-spoken man, speaks in clipped sentences. Tall and gracious, he gestured out the windows of the office where we talked, at the elegant old buildings across the street that house Berklee's ever-expanding needs, taking over an old hotel, a theater.

He seems happy in his adjusted career, happy in his marriage and his life. He mentioned his wife and three children several times. His oldest child, Ben, is the composer of "Turn It to the Left," a rap video, available on YouTube, whose message is the danger of hearing loss from iPods and other personal listening devices. Ben is a lawyer, an amateur musician. Jackson's second child, Kate, works in finance, specializing in the fields of energy and health care. "My third child, Caroline," he told me with great pride, "interprets for the deaf. She's a certified interpreter. Sign language found her. She was eleven. Cleveland SoundStage [which performed skits about the deaf] came to her school, and she was fascinated that she could communicate with her hands. We're also a family interested in languages. So she had an underpinning. She's a healer and a communicator."

Jackson, too, is a communicator. It's very important, he said, that students know about his hearing loss. "In any orchestra there are people with hearing loss. The students need to understand this."

ELEVEN

The Ugly Stepsisters: Tinnitus and Vertigo

Hearing loss often is accompanied by two other conditions, both of which can be more debilitating than the hearing loss itself. The first is tinnitus and the second, which I have had several unfortunate experiences with and will discuss in the second half of the chapter, is vertigo.

Tinnitus is a sound in the ear or in the head with no known acoustic source, a "phantom sound." It is usually described as a ringing or buzzing, but it may also manifest itself as humming, whistling, ticking, a noise like crickets, roaring, falling water. The ethereal outer-space hum I hear is a form of tinnitus. Unusually, for someone with severe hearing loss, mine does not come often and is not especially bothersome.

Tinnitus is surprisingly common, a chronic condition affecting between 30 and 50 million Americans. Millions of others experience it from time to time. In a fraction of the chronic cases, about 5 percent, tinnitus is the result of physiological problems such as an acoustic neuroma, a eustachian tube dysfunction, and other medically or surgically treatable conditions. This type is referred to as objective tinnitus, and a doctor can hear it, using the right equipment. The other 95 percent suffer subjective tinnitus, which can be heard only by the sufferer.

Subjective tinnitus typically accompanies sensorineural hearing loss, whether of unknown etiology or caused by aging or noise exposure. It also occasionally occurs in people with normal hearing. About half of those affected are bothered by the noise. In 10 to 20 percent, the tinnitus is considered a "clinically significant condition." One percent of those with tinnitus report that it substantially affects their quality of life. Tinnitus is difficult to measure using objective tests and is often rated on a scale from "slight" to "catastrophic."

The ongoing MarkeTrak studies focused in November 2011 on tinnitus. Kochkin's co-authors were Richard Tyler, a professor at the University of Iowa who has edited three books on tinnitus, and Jennifer Born, director of public affairs at the American Tinnitus Association. Their study excluded people living in nursing homes and other institutions. They found tinnitus increases with age, affecting as many as 26.7 percent of people aged sixty-five to eighty-four.

Surprisingly, the survey found that 13 million people reported that they had tinnitus but not hearing loss. Researchers think that tinnitus accompanies hearing loss in by far the majority of cases, and the authors suggest that the tinnitus these people have may be masking their hearing loss. If that is the case, it would mean that the numbers for those with hearing loss would increase substantially, from 36 million to 47.5 million—very close to the 2011 figures from Johns Hopkins.

The study found that almost 25 percent of those with tinnitus describe it as disabling or nearly disabling. In general, the greater the degree of hearing loss, the louder the tinnitus. "In severe cases," the Kochkin report said, "it can interfere with the individual's ability to perform adequately on the job or contribute to psychological disorders, such as depression, suicide ideation, post-traumatic stress disorder, anxiety and anger. The constancy of tinnitus and the perceived lack of control can provoke fear, which exacerbates the problem leading to an ever increasing cycle of distress in the person suffering from tinnitus."

Tinnitus is subjective in another sense as well: it may drive one person crazy and be waved away as an irritation by another. The response to tinnitus seems in some ways tied to the personality of the sufferer. A 2004 article by Robert A. Dobie (which appears in *Tinnitus: Theory and Management* by James Byron Snow) cited a 1988 study (of which he was a co-author) that found that most patients with "really bothersome" tinnitus also had a major depressive disorder. About half of depressed tinnitus patients, he went on, reported that their depression preceded tinnitus. "It seems likely that people who have had prior problems with depression, and possibly with anxiety disorders, are more likely to become tinnitus sufferers than are people who have not had such problems."

Anecdotally, tinnitus has been linked to suicide: Former Greene County (Virginia) Sheriff William L. "Willie" Morris left a note saying he was killing himself because of the constant roar in his ears. A British rock fan stabbed himself to death three months after developing tinnitus at a live concert by the U.S. group Them Crooked Vultures.

A 2001 study of the scientific literature between 1966 and 2001 found "no cause and effect relationship between tinnitus and suicide." The study, published in the *Journal of the American Academy of Audiology*, concludes: "More often, patients who had attempted or committed suicide had significant preexisting psychiatric conditions, the most common being depression. Accordingly, it is our conclusion that nowhere in the existing literature is there any evidence supporting a cause and effect relationship between tinnitus and suicide." Dobie agrees, noting a study of 287 patients with tinnitus who had committed suicide. "Most were male, elderly, socially isolated, and depressed—classic warning signs for suicide with or without tinnitus."

Despite the subjective experience of tinnitus, it has a physiological cause. Research has found that when hearing loss occurs, there is usually damage to the auditory receptors, the hair cells. This leads to a loss of normal function in the auditory nerve, which itself leads to loss of normal input to the neurons throughout the auditory system of the brain. The neurons are connected by synapses, some of which are excitatory (causing activity to increase) and some of which are inhibitory (reducing the level of activity). These synapses are out of whack, causing spontaneous activity in the neurons, which tinnitus sufferers hear as noise. Tinnitus is especially associated with high-frequency noise-related hearing loss, which may explain why tinnitus is often pitched at a high frequency.

• • •

Tinnitus has a long history. The earliest undisputed description of tinnitus comes from Hippocrates, according to Jerome Groopman, who suffers from tinnitus himself and who wrote about it in *The New Yorker* in 2009. Hippocrates described the noises as *echos* (sound), *bombos* (buzzing), and *psophos* (a slight sound). The word "tinnitus" derives from the Latin word *tinnire*, to ring.

The list of people known or suspected to have had tinnitus is, as might be expected, very long. Here are just a few:

Darwin: Tinnitus was the least of it. As he described in a letter summarizing his health to a new doctor in 1865:

> Age 56–57.—For 25 years extreme spasmodic daily & nightly flatulence: occasional vomiting, on two occasions prolonged during months. Vomiting preceded by shivering, hysterical crying, dying sensations or half-faint. & copious very palid urine. Now vomiting & every paroxys[m] of flatulence preceded by singing of ears, rocking, treading on air & vision. focus & black dots—All fatigues, specially reading, brings on these Head symptoms ?? nervousness when E[mma] leaves me . . .

Van Gogh: There is speculation that tinnitus drove him to cut off his ear before he committed suicide.

Beethoven: In 1801, when he was thirty-one, he wrote in a letter to a friend that his hearing had grown steadily weaker over the past three years. "In the theatre I have to get very close to the orchestra to understand the performers, and that from a distance I do not hear the high notes of the instruments and the singers' voices." He noted that he couldn't hear quiet voices, adding, "The sound I can hear it is true, but not the words," a sensation familiar to many with hearing loss, as is the next sentence: "If anyone shouts I can't bear it." He also suffered from tinnitus, "rushing and roaring sounds" in his head. A December 2011 article in the *British Medical Journal* speculated that Beethoven's high-frequency hearing loss may have affected his middle-period music, which used fewer high notes than his early or late period (when he was completely deaf). Jay Alan Zimmerman has also written on Beethoven's hearing loss and its effect on his music, from the perspective of a fellow composer: in an article intended for the *Canadian Hearing Report* he wrote:

> The overwhelming trend in Beethoven's music of this period is a slow stretch of melody to its lowest possible extremes, followed by a reduction in its highest. He moves from open chords in the low register to thick triads. And though the new, modern piano has extra high notes, he focuses instead on its ability to express a darker, louder, dynamic range.
>
> Did this lowered "pitch shift" occur: Accidentally—as a part of his desire to create a darker, more emotional style of music than the Classical Era? Subconsciously—as a result of his losing the ability to hear the high notes? Or, consciously—so that he could perform these pieces with more confidence?
>
> As a composer who's gone through this same stage while writing and performing my own works, my guess is: a combination of all three. Sometimes I "hide" low note cues in my work so that I can perform it. Sometimes I just want to enjoy hearing the music, so I write it in my hearing

range. And sometimes, frankly, I have no clue what I'm doing. It happens instinctively.

William Shatner and David Letterman: Shatner developed tinnitus after a prop explosion on the set of an episode of *Star Trek* in the mid-sixties. In a 1996 interview with David Letterman, he described hearing the ocean in his ears even when he was in the desert. Letterman described his own tinnitus as a combination of a hissing sound, "shhhhhh," and high-pitched "eeee"—"I'm testing the emergency broadcast system every minute of my life," he quipped. The interview was funny, with an undercurrent of desperation in both.

The list of pop musicians with tinnitus is lengthy and often overlaps with those with hearing loss: Pete Townshend, Neil Young (who switched to acoustic music to lessen the damage to his ears), Eric Clapton, Bono and The Edge, Moby, George Harrison. Will.i.am, of the Black Eyed Peas, says the only relief for his tinnitus is loud music. "I don't know what silence sounds like anymore. Music is the only thing which eases my pain," he told the British newspaper *The Sun* in 2010. Think of any of your favorite rock musicians from the seventies and eighties and some of them suffer from tinnitus. For many, music is the cause and music is the "cure," at least as long as it's masking the tinnitus. "I can't be quiet," Will.i.am said, "as that's when I notice the ringing in my ears. There's always a beep there every day, all day."

Tinnitus treatment has in some ways not become any more sophisticated than it was in Greco-Roman days. Then, Groopman tells us, it ranged from holding the breath "to expel offending humors" to placing honey, vinegar, cucumber juice, and radish extract in the ear. Current therapies aim not to reverse tinnitus but to make it bearable. The most common treatment—which is reversible if it doesn't work—is to fit the sufferer with hearing aids. Hearing aids both amplify background noise, masking the perception of tinnitus, and improve the patient's ability to communicate, resulting in a decrease in stress. This doesn't "cure" tinnitus, but as Robert A. Dobie, writing in the James Byron Snow book, said: "In my opinion, the success or failure of such treatments should be measured in terms of the reduction in suffering, not the change in sensation."

A special issue of *The Hearing Journal* (November 2010) focused on new approaches to treating tinnitus. In it, Robert W. Sweetow, a well-respected authority on tinnitus, wrote, "There are so many conflicting and unsubstantiated claims of so-called 'cures' or 'treatments' found in the professional literature, the Internet, and the mainstream media in ubiquitous advertisements that hearing healthcare professionals must be vigilant both in the pursuit of better management procedures and in critically evaluating 'evidence' in an unbiased and scientific manner."

Indeed, the profusion of novel and often unscientific approaches to the treatment of tinnitus at first made Sweetow hesitant about accepting the guest editorship—for fear, he said, of providing "a forum for promoting treatments that have little or no evidence base." As a further caveat, he added, "The inclusion of an article in this special issue should not be interpreted as an endorsement of the approach it discusses by either me, as guest editor, or *The Hearing Journal*."

The theories offered fell into four general approaches to tinnitus management.

Acoustic management, in which the use of temporally patterned sounds—"cortically interesting sounds"—may alter abnormal activities to suppress tinnitus. Other papers discussed masking and sound-enrichment techniques that go beyond those now being used.

Papers on pharmacological management advocated for a multidisciplinary approach (including the use of anti-insomnia medications, benzodiazepines, and antidepressants). "Patients experiencing severe tinnitus deserve the compassion and attention of their audiologist and primary-care clinician along with other specialists as needed. The uncertainty attached to having severe tinnitus along with the etiologic ambiguity is highly stressful," the author wrote. "The well-being of patients with severe tinnitus depends on seamless communication between the audiologist and the primary-care clinician. It is of utmost importance to replace a delayed and disjointed healthcare response with one that effectively diminishes tinnitus suffering and softens the impact of a chronic condition affecting millions."

Other pharmacological suggestions included the use of a ginkgo biloba–based treatment called Arches and another called Ring Stop, and a widely advertised homeopathic treatment called Quietus. As Sweetow said, "The inclusion of an article in this special issue should not be interpreted as an endorsement . . ."

Behavioral therapies proposed include "mindfulness-based" tinnitus therapy, an eight-week course based on Buddhist meditative practices but "without the Buddhism," writes Jennifer J. Gans of the University of California, San Francisco. Comparing mindfulness-based therapy to cognitive behavioral therapy, the author says they differ in almost mirror-like ways. Whereas CBT "is thought to increase realistic, logical, and rational thinking, which is thought to relieve distress and reduce maladaptive behaviors," mindfulness-based approaches "attempt to alter the perception of experiences in a kind, accepting, and non-judgmental manner. This change in perception is thought to facilitate coping flexibility, self-regulation, and clarification of values, and may even act as a form of exposure that results in reduction of stress."

That same issue also included a critique of repetitive transcranial magnetic stimulation, in which magnetic pulses are delivered repetitively and rhythmically, usually for thirty minutes, once a day for three to ten consecutive days. Results are mixed. Some sufferers have found relief for six months, others for only a few days to a few weeks. Several clinical trials of the technique are under way.

Not mentioned in the *Hearing Journal* issue but discussed

by Groopman are a few other remedies that desperate tinnitus sufferers may turn to: the neti pot, which is used to irrigate the nasal passages with warm salt water. And "ear candling." "People actually take wax paper, roll it up, stick one end in the ear canal, and light the other end."

It's no wonder that researchers—and patients—are willing to try anything. As Sweetow writes of current common procedures, the majority of tinnitus sufferers do not have "curable" tinnitus. "The next best course of action" is to address the auditory, attentional, and emotional issues attending to tinnitus.

Management strategies currently in use are Tinnitus Retraining Therapy, which uses a combination of counseling and auditory therapy—in the form of low-level sound—to teach the brain not to react to the stimulation as a threat. Retraining the brain to sort out meaningful from irrelevant stimuli requires first that tinnitus no longer carry a negative emotional association.

A second management technique is acoustic desensitization, called Neuromonics treatment. Using an MP3 player, the patient listens to music adapted for his or her hearing threshold, and presented at a level just loud enough to interfere with the tinnitus perception. The program involves the patient's listening passively for two to four hours a day to induce relaxation and desensitization.

In conclusion, the *Hearing Journal* editors wrote in their introduction to the issue, none of these therapies constitute a "cure." Nevertheless, "it is unethical and immoral for audiologists or hearing aid dispensers to tell a tinnitus sufferer, 'There is nothing that can be done for you. Just learn to live with it.'" People with tinnitus say that in fact that may be the only ethical thing to say: as of now, there is no cure, and treatments don't work.

Meanwhile, as Jerome Groopman wrote in *The New Yorker*, total funding for tinnitus research has recently been as little as $3 million a year. That's not going to support much clinical investigation into a problem that plagues 30 to 50 million Americans and half the soldiers returning from Afghanistan and Iraq.

• • •

The other ugly stepsister is vertigo.

It was late February, about a year and a half after my implant. My husband was the guest speaker at a gala dinner at the august Metropolitan Club at Sixtieth Street and Fifth Avenue. The occasion was the one hundredth anniversary of the New York Psychoanalytic Society, which he had been invited to address because his novel *The Treatment*, about an eccentric Cuban psychoanalyst, was a favorite among those in the profession—despite the analyst's outrageous behavior.

Psychoanalysis is an endangered practice. In its classic form— four or five times a week, lying on the couch—it's simply too expensive and too time-consuming for most people. But psychoanalytic psychotherapy, a modified version, is still popular, especially on the Upper West Side of Manhattan. I was interested to see how these upholders of the tradition would celebrate this occasion, and I was curious to see what my own psychotherapist, a psychoanalyst by training, looked like out of her office, which had come to seem an extension of her person. I was also looking forward to dressing up and going somewhere elegant.

Unfortunately, that morning I had emergency root canal surgery. The doctor gave me a prescription for Vicodin and I went home and took a nap. My teeth hurt and I was exhausted from days of tooth pain and narcotics, but I enjoyed the cocktail hour—cocktail-less for me. (My therapist, by the way, looked just about the same as always.) Then we went in to dinner. The smoked salmon came and I had a bite.

The first thing that happens with vertigo is that your eyes go out of control. I couldn't seem to hold them in one place. The ball-room, a sea of round tables and analysts, started tilting, left and right. I said to Dan, "I'm dizzy. I have to get out of here." He took me firmly by the arm and led me the (fortunately short) distance to the door. Once out into the elegant foyer, where just minutes before cocktails and chatter had filled the room, I said, "I'm going to be sick," and promptly was. The unflappable staff of the Metropolitan Club grabbed a trash can and then a chair, as it was clear I couldn't stay on my feet. Even as I reeled and vomited into the trash can, I retained enough vanity to hope they didn't think I was drunk.

After about forty-five minutes, I felt steady enough to get to a taxi, escorted on either side by sturdy waiters, a plastic bag for emergencies in my hand. My daughter had come to take me home, since my husband had not yet given his talk, and I urged him to stay. At home, I took a meclizine (the anti-nausea drug given to me when I had the implant surgery) and fell into a sound sleep. For a horrible experience, it wasn't so bad. I determined never to take Vicodin again.

But it wasn't the Vicodin. Three days later, I was sitting on a bench in a Verizon store, waiting for the technician to bring back my faulty cell phone. Suddenly my eyes crossed and the room tilted. I keeled over into a semiprone position. Someone got me into a taxi. At home I took a meclizine and slept. Over the next six weeks I had attacks every three or four days, lasting forty-five minutes to an hour. Afterward I would be exhausted and sleep, usually until the next morning. Most occurred when I was sitting still. At my computer, in a doctor's waiting room, reading, at dinner. I couldn't predict when an episode would occur. There seemed to be no common thread. Dr. Hoffman put me on Valium, which depresses the central nervous system and can help stave off episodes. It made my legs feel like logs and I went on having vertigo. He switched me to Klonopin, half a milligram twice a day. I eventually reduced it to half that, at my therapist's suggestion.

I had a balance test—an ENG, or electronystagmography, which the Vestibular Disorders Association describes as a "battery" of eye-movement tests, and it does feel like a battering. It's an elaborate production involving heavy goggles that hurt my nose, and a moving chair. During the tests the technician moved my head from side to side, while I kept my eyes open inside the darkened goggles. In another test I followed an LED light with my eyes as it moved rapidly left and right or up and down. Eye movement is measured by electrodes placed on the skin or, as in my case, with an infrared video camera mounted inside the goggles (the test is then called videonystagmography, VNG). They skipped the astronaut test, in which you're strapped in the chair and it turns upside down. The results were normal, "remarkably good," Dr. Hoffman said, considering that I have an implant. I also had a CT scan. Normal. That is, no explanation. Idiopathic.

Again I found myself asking "Why?" The most common form of vertigo—as opposed to dizziness or balance problems—is BPPV (benign paroxysmal positional vertigo). My sister has it. She describes it as coming on slowly, or as a result of getting up too quickly in the morning. It can also be brought on by prolonged time in a dentist's chair with your head back. A physical therapist can teach you exercises to prevent it. The technician who did my balance test said the vertigo I was having was not BPPV, though I think I have had it. Once, after lying on my back doing Pilates, I stood up and crashed into a mirror. An infection can also cause vertigo, often very severe but brief. A friend was hospitalized with vertigo a few years ago, and has never experienced an episode since.

Other potential causes include labyrinthitis (an inflammation of the inner ear—my inner ear was fine), acoustic neuroma (a benign growth on the vestibular nerve—the CT scan ruled that out), migraine in the form of vertigo (my episodes didn't seem to fit the description). That brought us back to Ménière's disease.

I never understood what true vertigo was until I had it. I transferred my obsession with the why of hearing loss to the why of vertigo. I found a kindred spirit in John Carey of Johns Hopkins. His enthusiasm for creative ways of diagnosing and treating vertigo was matched only by my own desire for just such solutions.

He described what happens in vertigo as if he were observing himself having an episode. "I have these rotation centers in my head and normally when my head is still, the neurons to these cells are firing equally from the two sides. If I turn to the left the right goes down, and vice versa. The reflex between the inner ear and turning your eyes is only seven milliseconds, the shortest reflex time in the body. You turn your head and your eyes start to compensate for that movement." He paused as if contemplating the brilliance of human anatomy. "You can't see seven milliseconds. But you can measure it." It's not just humans who have this reflex. "The inner ear, the balance part," he went on, "is important in all species. It keeps our eyes on target. Vestibular reflexes affect the visual system."

He told me about various standard and experimental efforts to treat vertigo caused by Ménière's. Even if I don't have classic Ménière's (I have only mild tinnitus and rarely a feeling of fullness in the ear, two of the four major symptoms), my vertigo probably is caused by a similar mechanism and may respond to similar efforts to control it.

As with many conditions, prevention starts with diet. "Restricted sodium may reduce vertigo attacks. But you have to really reduce it," Carey said. "FDA recommendations are now 1500 mg of salt a day." I pointed out that a Starbucks turkey sandwich contains about that amount of sodium. Exactly the problem, Carey agreed. Fifteen hundred mg a day is considered pretty low, and as the Starbucks sandwich shows, it's hard to achieve. Nevertheless, it's frequently not low enough to have an effect on vertigo, he said, "so often you add a diuretic—dyazide or the hydrochlorothiazides."

Too much caffeine or nicotine may reduce the blood flow to the inner ear (that's controversial), which may set off the chain of events leading to dizziness or vertigo. Stress and anxiety can exacerbate it, though not cause it. I suspected the Klonopin worked for me because it reduced anxiety, not because it had any direct effect on my vestibular system. I was reluctant to give it up. I had enough anxiety in my life without adding the anxiety about having another vertigo attack.

I found a number of blogs devoted to vertigo—Vertigo Guy, Dizzy Dame—writers whose suffering far outweighs mine. Vertigo Guy has tried everything, including Vestibular Rehab Therapy— a long-term treatment to help train your eyes to adjust to vertigo-inducing situations. Often it makes the vertigo worse before (and sometimes instead of) making it better. Vertigo Guy also tried the BrainPort, a device that gives a shock to your tongue when you go off-center. You wear it for twenty minutes a day. Last time Vertigo Guy blogged, it didn't seem to be working.

John Carey was one of the authors of a 2007 retrospective study of the use of dexamethasone, a steroid injected through the eardrum, as a treatment for vertigo in Ménière's disease. The study group was 129 patients at Hopkins who had unilateral Ménière's disease and had not responded to changes in diet or the use of diuretics. The results, though retrospective (which is less desirable than prospective), were persuasive. A hundred and seventeen, or 91 percent, found that the dexamethasone treatment controlled their vertigo. Thirty-seven percent required just one injection, 20 percent responded after two, 14 percent after three, and 8 percent after four. There was typically a three-month interval between injections.

The twelve patients who did not respond to treatment decided to try a more aggressive treatment with injected gentamicin, an antibiotic that, ironically, damages the hair cells of the inner ear that are responsible for balance function. I asked John Carey why *damaging* balance hair cells could help in Ménière's disease. It gets to the point of the problem in Ménière's, says Carey: "The problem isn't the loss of inner ear balance function. It's the unpredictable spells in which the balance function goes haywire—the balance nerve on one side starts firing faster than it should." The hair cells govern the nerve's firing, so taking out some of these cells seems to lessen the chance of the nerve's firing going haywire.

The other side of the gentamicin sword is that it does decrease some of the hearing in the ear being injected. "Our research suggests that gentamicin damages a fraction of the hair cells—the so-called type I cells—of the inner ear, but doesn't damage the nerve. Although the ability to sense some rapid head movements decreases after gentamicin treatment, patients generally find the relief of so much greater benefit that it is worth it. The loss of function is less than what we get with surgeries that destroy function—labyrinthectomy or vestibular nerve section." Because gentamicin can also damage hearing hair cells, the number of injections is usually carefully controlled to cause "just enough" loss of balance function to stop the attacks.

Carey said no one knew why the dexamethasone worked. "It could be an anti-inflammatory, or it could regulate the sodium, which also results in the feeling of fullness in the ear and in tinnitus." In the end, although it can control vertigo, it cannot cure Ménière's disease. In their paper, the authors suggest that intratympanic dexamethasone treatment may simply provide temporary relief until spontaneous remission of the vertigo occurs. This happens in about 70 percent of cases of Ménière's disease, usually leaving some permanent hearing and balance function loss.

I had only mild vertigo for a few months after I started on Klonopin. Then, one summer afternoon at a friend's swimming party, I had another attack, a bad one. I staggered out of the pool area, threw up on the lawn, and lay down on the grass for an hour or so before my friend arranged for someone to drive me home. She proved to be a regular Florence Nightingale, bringing me a towel to lie on, offering me water from time to time, asking if I was okay, but basically leaving me to sleep it off. Dr. Hoffman added a tiny dose of Elavil, an antidepressant usually given in minimum doses of 150 mg. He prescribed 10 mg, once a day. This plus the Klonopin again worked for a while.

In December, shopping for Christmas presents for my children, I went into the vibrant new Uniqlo store on Fifth Avenue, up the two-story-long escalator, into a maze of clothing racks and counters. This time the only way out was by ambulance. Now I take half a Klonopin and 20 mg of Elavil every night and half a Klonopin and two Advils every morning. So far, so good.

My internist sent me to a neurologist to see if my vertigo might be migraine-induced. He did some tests to see if some kind of arterial blockage might be the cause. He found some mild blockage but not enough to cause vertigo, and agreed with Dr. Hoffman that if the drug regimen was working, don't mess with it. The only side effect of the drugs is that I sleep eight deep hours a night, a bonus for a lifelong insomniac. Sometimes I even take a mid-afternoon nap. The rest of the time I feel fine. But like many people, I have an irrational objection to taking so many drugs. Are they really working? Maybe it's gone away on its own. The temptation to stop the drugs and see what happens is strong, but not strong enough yet to overcome the memory of what it feels like to have vertigo.

VOICES: MELISSA

"My vertigo 'episode' lasted for about six weeks," Melissa (who asked that her last name be omitted) wrote to me. "It was an awful experience; vomiting, crawling to get to the bathroom, looking like a drunkard at any time of day, all of which created the ongoing day-to-day isolation and depression that come with illness and job loss.

"After six weeks of being homebound (flat on the floor), I was able to slowly start physical therapy. I saw a specialist in vestibular disorders. Now it is hard for me to believe that I could not step over a shoebox without falling to the ground, or walk down the narrow hallway without bumping off of the walls."

Melissa is a neighbor of my sister, Jean, in Seattle. One day when Jean and I were out walking her dog, we ran into Melissa. Despite her assurance that she was up and well, it was still a surprise to find her a robust, tanned, and almost hyperenergetic woman. She had just come back from Honduras, where she had been snorkeling and swimming and kayaking.

The following morning I joined Melissa in her daily three-mile walk, up and down the hills above the University of Washington campus. She walked so fast I had to run to keep up as she told me her horrific story. The vertigo episode had happened seven years before, she told me. She was folding laundry, bent over to pick something up, and hit the floor. Her hearing and balance were gone. After her doctor determined that she had not had a stroke or any other medical condition that could have caused the vertigo, she began a grueling series of exercises to compensate for the vertigo and "create a new normal," as she put it.

The exercises themselves caused vertigo and so had to be done in a quiet private space. She had physical therapy, practiced tai chi, used an exercise bike, practiced yoga, lifted weights. And she walked, for some time with a cane, accompanied by her husband. She went on a low-salt, low-fat diet, drank wine only in moderation, and took Valium when she felt an attack coming on. She had also lost the hearing in her left ear, and eventually she got a bone-anchored implant (a BAHA made by Cochlear) in that ear, which allows her to hear "absolutely nothing," but helps her with perceiving sounds and maintaining her balance.

Her doctors have found no explanation for the vertigo and hearing loss. She has several allergies and thinks she may have an undetected autoimmune disorder. She's philosophical about the experience: she misses many things, she says, and social situations are particularly challenging, but, she added, "at least I can be active and have learned to be at peace with myself." She was forced to slow down, but found "gifts" to compensate: meditation, drawing classes.

It's all been "a bit disturbing to one who likes to be—needs to be—in control," she wrote. "I certainly have given that up after this experience!"

TWELVE

Chicks and Fish Do It. Why Can't We?

"You'll never be deaf," Dr. Hoffman said to me years ago. At the time, I thought he meant I'd never lose all my hearing. But what I know now is that technology would take over when my ears no longer worked. Through a cochlear implant, I would continue to hear long after my ears ceased to function.

Research holds the promise that the kind of hearing loss I have may someday be reversible, returning the ear to close to its original pristine condition. Probably not soon and not for me, but most researchers think that within a decade they may have the tools that will eventually allow doctors to stop the progression of sensorineural hearing loss, including age-related hearing loss. Putting those tools into practice will take much longer. (Gene therapy, for people whose hearing loss has a genetic basis, will probably come sooner, possibly in the next decade.) The best guesses for hair cell regeneration—for the much larger group of people whose sensorineural loss is caused by noise or ototoxins or age—range anywhere from twenty to fifty years.

Until recently, scientists focused on the development of devices that would take the place of normal hearing: hearing aids and cochlear implants. The pharmaceutical industry, usually so quick to jump on the opportunity to medicalize a chronic age-related condition—dry eyes and wrinkles, trouble sleeping, lagging sexual function, bladder control, memory loss—has not paid much attention to age-related hearing loss, in terms of either prevention or cure. There are no FDA-approved drugs for the treatment of hearing loss. Demographics alone would suggest they are missing a big opportunity.

In October 2011, the Hearing Health Foundation (formerly the Deafness Research Foundation) held a symposium in New York to kick off its new campaign, called the Hearing Restoration Project, an ambitious program that had enlisted, at that point, fourteen researchers from ten major hearing loss research centers in the United States. This consortium will share findings, with the goal of developing a biological cure for hearing loss in the next ten years. With a fund-raising target of $50 million, or $5 million a year, the Hearing Restoration Project will tackle the problem of hearing loss with the aim of curing it, rather than simply treating it.

The funding is relatively small right now, but there is hope that the foundation will be able to raise more in future years. Individual consortium members may currently receive somewhere between 5 and 20 percent of their laboratory's annual budget from the Hearing Health Foundation. But the collaborative nature of the venture is unusual. (A similar consortium exists for the study of myelin diseases—a factor in multiple sclerosis as well as hereditary neurodegenerative diseases.) Under its previous name, the Deafness Research Foundation, funding was limited to researchers in the early years of their careers. They've now added the Hearing Restoration Project.

The symposium, titled "The Promise of Cell Regeneration," brought together leading researchers in the field of hearing loss. Dr. George A. Gates, an M.D. and the scientific director of the Hearing Restoration Project, chaired the program. The speakers included Sujana Chandrasekhar, an M.D. and director of New York Otology, who talked from a clinical perspective about the current state of hearing loss research. Ed Rubel, from the University of Washington, discussed the history of hair cell regeneration research and his current work on regenerating hair cells through pharmaceutical applications. Stefan Heller discussed his lab's announcement in May of 2010 of the first successful attempt at generating mammalian hair cells (of mice) in a laboratory setting from stem cell transplants. Andy Groves, from Baylor, discussed the many still-existing hurdles to hair cell regeneration in humans. Unable to attend was Douglas Cotanche, currently working at Harvard on noise-induced hearing loss in military personnel.

Humans have 30,000 cochlear and vestibular hair cells. By contrast, the human retina has 120 million photoreceptors. The 30,000 hair cells, arranged in four rows and protected by the hard shell of the cochlea, determine how well you can hear. If you lose the outer cells, you suffer up to a 60-decibel hearing loss. That degree of hearing loss can usually be corrected with a hearing aid. If you lose the inner row of cells, you may have a total loss. The more inner cells damaged, the greater the degree of loss. Sharon Kujawa, speaking at the 2011 HLAA meeting, had described the damaged cells as lying flat, like a field of wheat after a storm. Stefan Heller drew an even more graphic picture of severe damage. The flattened cells, he said, may be "followed by a collapse of the tunnel of Corti, resulting in a structure that often features an unorganized mound of inconspicuous cells."

Surrounding the inner and outer hair cells are the so-called supporting cells, which come in all varieties: Deiters' cells, Claudius' cells, Hensen's cells, inner pillar and outer pillar cells. Supporting cells are the magical cells that instigate regeneration in damaged inner ears of chicks and fish. And they are where someday regeneration may occur in humans.

That limited number of hair cells, as well as their fragility and inaccessibility, has hampered research. In his 2010 *Cell* paper, Stefan Heller noted, "The inner ear shelters the last of our senses for which the molecular basis is unknown." So little is known about the structure of the inner ear that, as Dr. Gates said, "we have a hard time clinically knowing how much [loss] is outer and how much is inner. That's why we use the term 'sensorineural.'"

• • •

Ed Rubel's photo on the University of Washington website shows a balding middle-aged man, elbows on the table, with two yellow chicks. That whimsical photo belies a seriously impressive academic c.v.: Virginia Merrill Bloedel Professor of Hearing Science; Professor of Otolaryngology—Head and Neck Surgery; Professor of Physiology and Biophysics; Adjunct Professor of Psychology. Dr. Gates referred to him as the godfather of hair cell regeneration.

Rubel and his colleagues at the Virginia Merrill Bloedel Hearing Research Center see four clinical scenarios that lend themselves to pharmaceutical fixes. The first would reverse sudden sensorineural hearing loss. The second would prevent ototoxic and/or noise-related hearing loss. The third would retard the progression of hearing loss, especially age-related hearing loss. The fourth would restore hearing after it had been lost.

Until 1985 it was thought that no animals could regenerate hair cells once they were destroyed. Rubel, then at the University of Virginia, discovered, quite inadvertently, that some do. The purpose of his research was to determine how long it took for ototoxic drugs to damage hair cells. He and his lab partners chose chicks as their animal model. Chicks have an easily accessible inner ear, and their ears in many ways resemble the human inner ear.

Rubel gave the chicks hair-cell-destroying aminoglycocides—a class of antibiotic known to be ototoxic—and then assigned the new guy at the lab, as Rubel put it in his talk at the conference, a resident named Raul Cruz, to sacrifice the chicks after a certain number of days and study the degree of deterioration in the hair cells. After eight days, Cruz found the chicks had, as expected, lost many cells. But when he studied the slides taken from chicks sacrificed at twenty-two days, instead of more dead cells they showed fewer. Where there had been dead cells, there were now healthy ones. "Raul, you must have mixed up your animals, go back and do it again," Rubel recounted, adding, to laughs, "Because he was just a resident, he didn't know what he was doing."

Again, Cruz brought similar data. This time Rubel told him to change his counting criteria. Even then, the regenerated cells were still there. "Well, maybe I better look in the microscope," Rubel said. Cruz was right, of course. But no one understood the mechanism. "What's going on here?" they asked themselves.

Around the same time, Doug Cotanche, then a postdoc at the University of Pennsylvania, saw the same results in chicks after damage due to intense noise exposure. Rubel and Cotanche published separate papers in different scientific journals, but continued communicating and soon got together to publish dual papers in the prestigious journal *Science*, showing, as Rubel said, that these were indeed brand-new hair cells "due to new cell division and the creation of new cells in the inner ear." This was a stunning scientific development. "And wow, we had a new field."

The next step was to figure out how chickens did it. Studying the cochlea of chicks and other birds, Rubel and others found eventually—over eighteen years!—that bird hair cells do indeed regenerate. Over the same period they discovered many other important molecular and functional details related to this remarkable ability. He showed some slides. The first slide showed the condition of the hair cells shortly after the animals were exposed to noise: "It looks just terrible. All these hair cells are blebbing out and being discarded." Five days later, however, they could see "baby cells" budding, some of them with the distinctive hair, or microvillus, on top. Then, after a few days, a high-power scanning electron microscope showed that all the hair cells were back. Not perfect, a few small abnormalities, but perfectly functional.

Interestingly, Rubel went on, they found that this happened no matter the age of the bird. Brenda Ryals, a former student of Rubel's, had a colony of senile quail that, they found, "regenerate cells just as well as a baby chicken does," Rubel said. New cells are created not only in the cochlea but also in the vestibular epithelium, important for balance. And, perhaps most important, the new cells are appropriately connected to the brain. "The new cells restore near-normal hearing and perfectly normal vestibular reflexes. They restore perception and production of complex vocalizations. Birds lose their song when they lose their hearing, but they gain their song back when they restore their hearing."

In 2001, Rubel joined forces with David Raible, also at UW, who was using zebrafish, a popular aquarium species, to study development of the nervous system. Eleven years later, the two labs are still collaborating on understanding how to prevent and cure hearing loss, and on hair cell regeneration.

Zebrafish proved to be an even better animal model than birds for studying some aspects of hearing loss prevention and regeneration. In addition to hair cells in the inner ear, aquatic vertebrates like fish have hair cells on the outside of the body, in something called the lateral line. The lateral line is used for detecting change in water currents and its cells are physiologically very similar to human inner ear cells. At electron microscope level, intracellular structure is similar. It turns out that fish and reptiles, like birds, regenerate hair cells, as do frogs and other animals. "So why can't we?" Rubel asked.

The Rubel/Raible team subjected the zebrafish larvae to ototoxic screening, again using aminoglycoside antibiotics. They tested drugs and druglike compounds to find ones that inhibit hair cell death in the fish. This work may lead to the development of protective cocktails to preserve hair cells before exposure to antibiotics or ototoxic chemotherapy drugs. They may also be given to humans after ototoxic assaults, which include noise exposure.

So far, testing on mammals, not to mention humans, is preliminary. Each human cochlea has only those 15,000 hair cells (the other 15,000 are in the vestibular system), and they are inaccessible in a living person. These generally decrease as we age, although not always. "Some animals and some humans seem resistant to noise and drugs and some humans hear perfectly until old age," Rubel said. "What grants this protection? Do some people have genetically 'tough' ears and others have 'weak' ears? If so, what are the genes responsible for this difference, and can we use them to protect hearing?" By doing genetic screening in zebrafish, it may be possible to find these genes and then find the cellular pathways to turn "weak ears" into "tough ears."

In March of 2012, I met with Rubel and a group of younger fellow researchers at the Virginia Merrill Bloedel center. Rubel is a charismatic leader, but he insisted on referring to these researchers not as part of his lab but as independent scientists, with their own NIH grants, some with their own hearing restoration projects. David Raible was out of town. Raible, Jennifer Stone, and Elizabeth Oesterle collaborate on different projects with each other and with Rubel. But, Rubel said, "Having sort of started the hair cell regeneration field, I feel very comfortable getting out of it and doing other things."

Jennifer Stone is a cell biologist and neuroanatomist who works primarily on avian hair cell regeneration. About five or six years ago she started working with mice, with several of the other participants, including Rubel and Elizabeth Oesterle, a cell biologist, and Clifford Hume, an M.D./Ph.D. clinician scientist. Stone led a recent study which found that after virtually all the vestibular hair cells in adult mice are killed, 16 percent of the hair cell population comes back spontaneously.

"It's a new discovery," Stone said. "It's not entirely surprising, but I think we've demonstrated it pretty definitively." Because spontaneous regeneration happens in only certain regions of the vestibular system, it helps the researchers narrow the field. By comparing the tissue in this region to tissue in others, they may understand the factor that allows regeneration in one place but not in another. Once we understand what allows the tissue to make new hair cells in these regions, Stone said, we can determine what would be needed to "release the brake," as she put it.

The p27 gene, which regulates cell division and helps prevent cancer, is one such molecule. To allow these hair cells to divide, the p27 gene would need to be turned off. Or maybe, she added, "it could be that we need to push the pedal on the gas: add something to promote division. It could be that we have to both put on the brakes and push on the pedal to start this process in mammals."

Julian Simon is a chemist, a Ph.D. pharmacologist, who got interested in the toxicity of cancer therapeutic drugs when clinicians at the Seattle Cancer Care Alliance, the patient arm of the Fred Hutchinson Cancer Research Center and the University of Washington, complained about the ototoxicity of certain chemotherapy drugs, Cisplatin prominently among them. Simon said that 30 to 40 percent of patients who go on Cisplatin regimens for lung cancer sustain significant and permanent hearing loss. (Rubel told me that some reports suggest an even higher percentage, up to 80 percent.) Simon's approach is to use small molecules to "perturb" biological systems. "We know what we'd like the cells to do, and in this case we'd like to take cells that would otherwise die and keep them living." Because the whole process of sensory hair cell death is— "with all due respect to present company" (meaning his fellow researchers)—"poorly understood, by learning how we can protect these cells from dying, maybe we can also learn something about the way cells die. Why they die."

Clifford Hume and Henry Ou are clinicians. Ou is a pediatric otolaryngologist at Seattle Children's Hospital. Both split their time between clinical work and research. As Ou said, "I help families understand hearing loss, try to diagnose the cause of the hearing loss in their child. And I try to figure out the etiology of hearing loss in general—in both kids who develop it and kids who are born with it."

The team's approach is multidisciplinary, involving not only research scientists and clinicians but also psychologists, genetic counselors, audiologists, and special education specialists. In adult hearing loss, they are also looking at the role of prescription medications in age-related hearing loss. Many are lifesaving medications, but sometimes less toxic substitutes may be available.

The UW group moved on to a lively discussion about how they would advise the parents of a young child getting implants. Should the child get implants in both ears? Cochlear implants cause the destruction of the so-called support cells that might give rise to new hair cells. Hence, should the parents "save" one ear in the hope that cell regeneration technology will eventually enable the child to hear normally out of that ear? Henry Ou said that parents often ask him about a second implant. "Sometimes they ask, 'Do you think there's hope that this is going to be fixed?' I say, 'Yeah.' But at the same time, if I don't think there's hope, I shouldn't be doing research on it. I'm a conflicted person to ask."

Simon added: "Parents don't want to find out when their kid is eighteen that there is something better." He cited the substantial evidence that children do better in school when they're implanted earlier, and bilaterally. Rubel agreed with the basic premise that early intervention is enormously important and that cochlear implants in children have become an essential therapeutic option, but expressed skepticism about the value of always doing bilateral cochlear implant surgery. Referring to one study in particular, he said, "The little-known fact about this work is that it includes only the top 20 percent of single implant users." Another study found different results. "So I think it's still up in the air," Rubel said.

We just don't have enough information yet to know the impact that implants make at that critical learning period for language and speech comprehension. But, as Jenny Stone said, the same question could be asked about regenerated hair cells. "The big elephant in the room, I think," she said, "is that we don't know whether regenerated hair cells will result in better hearing—appreciation of music, noise, speech—than a cochlear implant can. And I think it's a huge jump to assume that in twenty years we'll be there."

"Well, but in fifty years?" Rubel interjected.

"Maybe in fifty years," Stone replied.

"I keep going back to the bird," Rubel said, "and we absolutely know that the bird gets great hearing back. They can recognize their own songs, they can learn new songs, not only speech but song recognition!"

"He loves birds," Jenny Stone said. "I'm not trying to be pessimistic. But it's going to take a lot of time to really get concrete evidence for what the best type of repair is going to look like."

• • •

How is it that mammals got shortchanged in the hair cell regeneration department? Birds and mammals split 300 million years ago. Birds share a more recent common ancestor with reptiles. The hair cells of a bird are "scattered in a mosaic all over the surface of the hearing organ," Andy Groves told the Hearing Restoration conference. Mammals, by contrast, have decreased the number of hair cells and specialized the function of the supporting cells surrounding them. Supporting cells physically position hair cells, Groves explained, and they provide structural integrity to the cochlea to make it mechanically sensitive.

Why would this evolutionary adaptation have occurred? Groves speculates that mammals made a trade-off: in the course of developing high-frequency hearing, their hair cells became more specialized, and in the process they lost the ability to regenerate. Although we humans have devised many ways of inflicting hearing loss on ourselves (such as rock concerts, iPods, and heavy machinery), one of the few naturally occurring things that kill hair cells is the wear and tear of old age. (Unless it turns out that even that is the result of accumulated noise exposure.)

"From an evolutionary point of view," Groves said, "and this sounds rather brutal, but evolution doesn't care about old age, as long as you live long enough to have kids." Once your reproductive years are over, your body has done its evolutionary job. As a result, mammals would not suffer a selective disadvantage by losing the capacity to regenerate their hair cells.

Bruce Tempel, at the University of Washington, echoed that Darwinian opinion. For the past twenty to twenty-five years he has been looking at the genes implicated at one or another level in hearing loss. "Truth be told," he said in an interview, "the reason that I got really interested in the auditory system is because you don't need it. From a geneticist's point of view, basically, this is great. This system can be completely nonfunctional and the animal still survives." He added that stress and hormonal influences on hearing loss are part of the reason the auditory system is so useful to geneticists: "You're able to identify the genes, the proteins, and from studying the protein itself find out whether there's a hormone or an influence on the expression of that protein. You can find out if there are interacting proteins that become a cascade linking the different individual proteins and the genes. And what's really cool about the auditory system is that we can do all that and still have a viable animal."

• • •

Andy Groves also studies the genetics of hearing loss. One of the mammalian genes whose function is to stop cells from dividing (necessary to regulate the size of organs and protect against cancer) is the p27 gene, which Jenny Stone talked about at the UW group meeting. Figuring out how to switch off that gene is one of the biggest obstacles researchers face.

After a great deal of work in cell-culture dishes and looking through microscopes, Groves and his colleague Neil Segil discovered that when they isolated mouse supporting cells from the newborn cochlea, the action triggered the p27 gene to switch off and the supporting cells to start dividing. They don't know why. Unlike humans, mice cannot hear when they are born. Once mice begin to hear—at about two weeks after birth—the supporting cells stubbornly refuse to divide even when isolated from the cochlea. Groves, Segil, and their colleagues are now trying to understand what happens to the aging supporting cells that makes them unable to divide.

How can supporting cells be coaxed into making more hair cells? Almost twenty years ago, it was proposed that hair cells and support cells, side by side, participate in an ongoing conversation using an evolutionarily ancient communication system called the Notch signaling pathway. The hair cell commands the support cell not to divide and prevents it from becoming a hair cell. Because the mammalian cochlea has evolved to have only four rows of cells, Groves explained, the creation of more cells would disrupt the mechanical properties of the cochlea, possibly preventing it from working properly.

The role of the Notch pathway in regulating the activity of the p27 gene is controversial. Groves mentioned work that Amy Kiernan, currently on the faculty at the University of Rochester, carried out when she was a postdoc with Tom Gridley at the Jackson Laboratory in Bar Harbor, Maine. She managed to inactivate the Notch signaling pathway in mice genetically. Her mice produced extra hair cells and showed some precocious cell division in the cochlea. Another researcher working with Groves and Segil, Angelika Doetzlhofer, did the same, using a pharmacological approach with drugs that blocked Notch signaling. When they blocked the signaling in newborn mice, they saw a 50 percent increase in hair cells and fewer supporting cells. These findings are preliminary, Groves cautioned, and the role of the Notch pathway is still being studied.

Following up on this, Groves and his colleagues repeated their Notch blocking experiments in older mice. By the time the mice were three days old, the increase in hair cells had dropped to 30 percent. In six-day-old mice, new hair cells were no longer produced. Although extrapolating this timetable to humans is tricky, the current data suggest that the human cochlea may no longer respond to Notch inhibitors by the time the fetus is five to six months old.

"So here is the take-home message," Groves concluded. "Our challenge—if you want to set a ten-year challenge—is to understand these roadblocks and then devise methods to get rid of them, and ultimately to apply these methods in a clinical setting." A clinical setting populated by humans. As Groves said at the beginning of his talk, "We're not here to treat hearing loss in birds."

• • •

Stefan Heller and his colleagues are taking a different approach to regenerating hair cells. They are attempting to get stem cells—undifferentiated cells that can develop into various specialized cells—to turn into hair cells, by mimicking the naturally occurring developmental processes that lead to formation of the inner ear. They do this in a culture dish and in a laboratory setting, which allows them to learn a lot about the process, such as what it actually takes to make sensory hair cells from scratch.

In March 2012, I visited Heller's lab at Stanford in Palo Alto. We literally ran into each other as I was looking for his office. Heller is formidably smart but completely unimposing in manner. He was wearing a well-worn T-shirt with a coffee cup on it (half full? half empty? "Definitely half full," he said), jeans, and sneakers. We talked in his office with a huge humming fish tank taking up about a sixth of the office. I asked if he had zebrafish. He said he didn't, but Dr. Robert Jackler, the chair of the Stanford Otolaryngology Department and the force behind the accumulation of brainpower that makes Stanford's one of the most important hearing research departments in the world, told me that Heller raises anemones to get novel fluorochromes for his research.

It had been two years since his article appeared in *Cell*, under the characteristically cryptic (to laymen) title: "Mechanosensitive Hair Cell–like Cells from Embryonic and Induced Pluripotent Stem Cells." As he had explained to the Hearing Restoration audience, his lab works with three kinds of stem cells. The first are embryonic stem cells, which are derived from the inner cell mass of a blastocyst, an early embryo. The lab uses both mouse embryonic stem cells and human embryonic stem cells. (In 2009, President Obama lifted an eight-year ban on federal funding of human embryonic stem cell research, vastly increasing the number of cells available to researchers. The cells are derived primarily from human embryos left after fertility treatments.) Dr. Heller noted that a scientist has to be really "talented" to grow these cells, which involve an underlying structure with other cells on top: if left on their own, they would overgrow everything. "This is quite a bit of maintenance. It's actually labor-intensive work."

The second type are the induced pluripotent stem cells (iPSCs) referred to in the title of the 2010 article. These are, according to the NIH website, "adult cells that have been genetically reprogrammed to an embryonic cell-like state." The NIH definition goes on: "It is not known if iPSCs and embryonic stem cells differ in clinically significant ways." That Heller and his lab were able to produce sensory hair cells in mice using both these kinds of stem cells is significant. Further, that they were "mechanosensitive" means that they were responsive to mechanical stimulation, and that these responses were similar to those in immature hair cells.

The third type are somatic stem cells, cells isolated from a specific organ—like the human ear. As attractive as these cells are to religious conservatives who oppose embryonic stem cell use, up until now they have not seemed to be a viable option because, as Heller said, "these cells are very rare."

Embryonic stem cells and pluripotent stem cells share an unfortunate feature: they can generate tumors. Heller said that he's received many e-mails from patients offering to be subjects for human trials. He showed the audience at the hearing regeneration conference a slide of a mouse that had been injected with a small number of these cells: "After one month, this mouse grows an enormous tumor." Before they can be used to regenerate hair cells, these stem cells will have to be rendered non-tumorigenic.

Somatic stem cells don't cause tumors, but there aren't enough of them. Scientists have not been able to isolate enough of these cells from the ear to study their advantages and disadvantages over the more abundant but problematic embryonic and pluripotent cells. Induced pluripotent stem cells appear to be the perfect compromise. These cells can be generated from virtually any cell of someone's body, and Heller's lab has been working with somatic cells derived from skin biopsies, usually from a patient's arm, a human patient with hearing loss.

"The work is very exciting," he told me. "Treating the cells from the biopsy with reprogramming factors, they can turn a somatic cell into an induced pluripotent stem cell (iPS cell). They can then grow them in a culture much the way they do embryonic cells, but without the religious or ethical controversy.

"We are basically making hair cells from human skin cells," he said. "These cells are not from the ear, so making the claim that these are hair cells is a difficult one. But they do have all the features of hair cells. They look like hair cells, they express genes that one would expect to find in hair cells, and they are functional, and moreover, we are approaching the point where we can generate human hair cells." Many steps remain before this becomes anything like a clinical reality, however, and each step takes a long time and a lot of money.

Just as a mouse embryo takes only three weeks to develop, compared to a human's nine months, the mouse embryonic stem cells take eighteen to twenty days to become hair cells. The human cells take forty. They require constant monitoring and tending, Heller said. "You can't just close the incubator and come back in a week and hope for the best. You have to—every day—replace the culture medium. You have to look at the cells. You have to clean out areas you don't like. It's a little bit like a garden. You're nurturing a very precious plant." The iPS cells have to reproduce for about thirty generations before they can be used for experiments, which means it takes about 150 days to successfully culture these cells from patients. By the spring of 2012, they had cultured biopsies from three patients with genetic hearing loss. They had funding for about twelve altogether, from the NIH.

It's a long way from mouse to man, but Heller said at the Hearing Restoration symposium that despite the challenge, "we're getting close."

One of the major findings of the past five or ten years, Heller said, is coming to understand the roadblocks. Once they know what obstacles stand in the way of transplantation, they can begin to figure out how to get around them. The first roadblock is the fact that these cells cause tumors. Looking ahead, Heller said, scientists need another five to ten years to solve that problem—a knotty one that involves learning how to generate pure cells and cells that are not tumorigenic. Once they solve that one, they will encounter new roadblocks: how to deliver the stem cells into the ear, how to determine the appropriate site for integration of cells, how to ensure their long-term survival, how to block immune system responses, how to make sure the cells function—"and, of course, whether the cells improve hearing."

As a young assistant professor, Heller told the Hearing Restoration symposium, if he had been asked how long it would take to cure hearing loss, he would have said, "You know, in five years we'll have a solution for certain things." Over time, he went on, "I got a sense of the difficulty of the problem and of all the roadblocks and the issues we have to deal with. And I'm getting frustrated myself [about] how long it takes to overcome a single one of these roadblocks. And then you're over one hill and there's another one." The difference now, he said, is that "we know where we have to go, and what we have to do. It's difficult to assess whether it will take ten years or twenty years or even fifty years."

Later, he went back to the time line again. "I think for transplantation we need another five to ten years before we are at the point where we can generate pure cells and cells that are not tumorigenic, to start doing experiments with animals."

Ed Rubel, in our interview, also gave a time line for his lab's work: "I think with proper funding, we can, in ten years, develop ways to get sufficient numbers of hair cells in a laboratory mammal cochlea as a model. We [meaning researchers in the field] will then go on to optimize the drug or drugs in all the ways needed to use them safely in humans, and only then go to clinical trials." He pointed out that they already know some genes and some compounds that facilitate the production of new hair cells under some conditions, but they don't have the lead compound. Even once they find that lead compound, he added, "all the safety trials, in vitro trials and small animal trials, all that preclinical work, usually takes eight to ten years."

As for gene therapy, for those whose hearing loss has a genetic basis, Stefan Heller cites what happened with research on vision and blindness: "Twenty years ago this was an open field, and now it has evolved into a flourishing clinical field and a very lively biotechnology field" with a market for drugs and procedures. "I think we can use the vectors and tools they've developed and bring them into our field. So I think five to seven years is probably a reasonable time frame for seeing results in animal studies. Gene therapy would be used on people whose deafness is caused by a mutation in a certain gene. If you could deliver the correct gene into the inner ear, you might be able to repair hearing loss before it progresses too far for repair.

"There are hurdles to overcome in this therapy as well: First, as always, safety concerns. Second, how to deliver the virus carrying the corrective gene into all the regions of the cochlea, that tiny inaccessible spiral. An injection that succeeds in getting only partway into the cochlea would leave the patient with middle- and low-frequency loss. To reach these areas might require opening the cochlea, which would carry a high risk of doing further damage. One further problem is ensuring that the hair cells grow where they are supposed to. Hair cells not at the correct location in the organ of Corti can themselves contribute to profound hearing loss."

As for the development of prophylactic drugs, the use of "high throughput methods" will help make the time line a little shorter. High throughput methods—also called high content screens—use multiple cell-culture dishes testing hundreds or thousands of compounds. Robots may also be used to speed the testing process. This requires work "with big pharma—because we cannot do this in our lab," Heller said. High throughput screening and the backing of big pharma would increase efficiency, allowing the earlier use of screens directly with human cells so they don't have to go through mice first and then on to humans.

. . .

The military is also on the front lines of hearing research, mostly in the development of hearing protection. Tinnitus is the number one service-connected disability for veterans receiving compensation. Hearing loss, which was number one from 1998 to 2005, is number two. In the decade ending in 2010, there were 840,865 service-related cases of tinnitus. Hearing loss affected 701,760. (These figures are for veterans of all wars.) Post-traumatic stress disorder was third, at 501,280.

For those veterans who claimed service-related disabilities in 2010, presumably most of them veterans of the Gulf War and Iraq and Afghanistan, tinnitus was still the leading disability, at 87,621, with hearing loss second at 60,229. Again, PTSD was third, at 42,679. These three accounted for almost a quarter of all service-connected disabilities, according to the Veterans Benefits Administration. Altogether, hearing-related disability for the period of the Global War on Terror is estimated at nearly 300,000. Tinnitus and hearing loss account for over 90 percent of impairments in the category called Impairment of Auditory Acuity, and each had been climbing for a decade at an annual rate of between 13 and 18 percent. In 2011, for the first time in a decade, Impairment of Auditory Acuity declined by 4.9 percent.

Lt. Col. Mark Packer is the executive director of a congressionally mandated DOD Hearing Center of Excellence, with headquarters at Lackland Air Force Base. He is also chief of Neurotology and Cranial Base Surgery in the San Antonio Military Health System, in San Antonio, Texas. We had an extended e-mail discussion about the military and hearing loss. Colonel Packer pointed out that although the claims mentioned above are all service-related claims, meaning that they are changes in the status of auditory function that occur during active-duty service, it's not possible to say what percent are battlefield injuries. A large part of the congressional mandate to the HCE is to develop a registry to track hearing loss and other auditory system injury.

For now, Colonel Packer notes, an accurate accounting is difficult for a number of reasons. Hearing loss is an invisible impairment, as noted elsewhere, a silent disability, and may not be immediately recognized, reported, or diagnosed. In addition, it may manifest as temporary threshold shift, with the damage not showing up until much later. Soldiers are reluctant to report hearing losses unless they are persistent or until they are bothered by loud ringing in the ear. They don't want to let their teammates down for such a "minor" problem. Sometimes fellow servicemen urge the injured soldier to seek help if the problem is obvious to them.

As an invisible impairment, hearing loss is a particularly insidious war wound, Colonel Packer noted. Because trauma teams may not recognize hearing impairment, the lack of communication and understanding can lead to delayed recovery and rehabilitation. Other wounds often take priority over hearing loss and ear injuries, and diagnosis requires the cooperation of the wounded soldier, which may not be possible because of concurrent brain injuries and altered mental states. Specialized equipment to measure hearing loss also may not be available.

Hearing protection is mandated in the military (the Global War on Terror is the first war for which this is the case), but hearing damage continues unabated. As Colonel Packer noted in a July 2011 publication, this is partly due to the paradox of the battlefield: "Hearing is a critical defense for the war fighter, warning against threat and danger and promoting self-preservation."

Hearing is an essential component of personal safety, and of communications between troops and commanders, he wrote. At the same time, troops need to be protected—not only from explosions and guns firing but from engines and machinery, armored vehicles, low-flying aircraft, "from the engines of mechanization of war."

How much is this costing? The Centers for Disease Control, calculating on the basis of self-reporting, found that 600,000 veterans in this period had suffered hearing loss or tinnitus. The CDC also found that veterans who served in the United States or overseas between September 2001 and March 2010 were four times likelier than nonveterans to have sensorineural hearing loss.

"Using a simple direct calculation of current compensation rates applied to all individual claims of hearing loss and tinnitus by degree of injury," the Veterans Benefits Administration stated, "2009 figures for Department of Veterans Affairs (VA) compensation benefits would be $976M for hearing loss and $920M for tinnitus." In fiscal year 2010, considering only major hearing loss disability, calculated compensations come to slightly more than $1 billion. For tinnitus the figure is $336 million. These total $1.39 billion for major auditory disabilities for the year.

These calculations are not so simple in reality, Colonel Packer said, noting that compensation rates are based on a constellation of injuries, with hearing impairment folded into the larger picture. Other direct and indirect costs to the military include the cost of hearing conservation programs; the cost of equipment damaged or lost as a result of hearing-loss miscommunication; the cost of hearing rehabilitation; and the cost of attrition, lost experience, retraining, replacement, education, and new recruitment to replace lost service members.

The Hearing Center of Excellence is expected to operate at full capacity by the end of 2013, contingent on the development of the hearing loss registry. It's a collaborative Department of Defense and Veterans Administration effort, with the Air Force as executive agent. It promotes outreach to academia, industry, and international partners. Although divisions of the Hearing Center of Excellence deal with prevention, clinical care, and research, the organizational concept is for the center to act as a virtual center integrating existing programs, identifying strengths and weaknesses in prevention and care, and identifying strategies to fill priority gaps. The overall result is expected to translate into better care, advocacy, and continuity for service members and veterans with hearing loss. The center will not provide care facilities or institute acoustic labs. Its goal is to reduce duplicative effort and provide the tools, transparency, and data management necessary for a coordinated effort.

The Defense Department has a long history of funding gaps in operational medicine and combat casualty care. Among the prophylactic measures the DOD has already put into effect is an earplug that uses a quick switch to turn the earplug to a higher protection level. In noisy environments that don't require acute listening—for instance, around helicopters or troop carriers—it can be switched to a closed or "constant protection" setting. The problem is getting the troops to actually use the earplugs. The Lackland Center mission includes education about the need for and proper use of hearing protection.

Another part of the mission at Lackland is a better definition of the noise environment and the development of devices both to enhance the ability to communicate and to preserve and protect hearing. For example, the Defense Department backed the development of a "hearing pill" seven or eight years ago. The compound, known as NAC, for N-acetylcysteine, is a nutritional supplement that helps the body produce more of the chemical glutathione, which helps defend hair cells against toxins. The Navy holds a patent on NAC for protection against hearing loss, and it licensed production to American BioHealth Group in San Diego.

Initially, it was thought the medication might reverse the effects of hearing loss from acoustic trauma. Ben J. Balough, a Navy captain and otolaryngologist at the Naval Medical Center San Diego, was leading research on the special formulation of N-acetylcysteine. The Navy conducted a double-blind, placebo-controlled clinical trial in 2004. The trial found that when compared to the placebo, NAC reduced permanent hearing loss in the ear closer to the source of acoustic trauma. NAC also showed potential in reversing other symptoms of acoustic trauma, such as tinnitus and balance disorders. The U.S. Department of Defense provided $2.5 million for more clinical trials, using higher dosing of NAC. A 2005 report in *The ASHA Leader* noted: "The Navy also is seeking to package the supplement in an actual pill form instead of previous formulation of an effervescent tablet mixed with water."

The result was BioHealth's "Hearing Pill," which for a time was available online for $19.95. In the end, the clinical results were not reproducible. But luckily, NAC doesn't seem to be the sole answer. Colonel Packer said there are several promising protective compounds in development, in collaboration with industry leaders.

The organizational efforts at Lackland are being extended to other congressionally mandated Centers of Excellence. The Hearing Center is leading the effort to develop integrated investigations with centers that deal with overlapping sensory injuries, including brain injury, vision loss, extremity injury, and chronic pain. Protective medicines that may improve function of one sense, Colonel Packer said, may improve function in others. The holistic model established by the Hearing Center can be applied to other leading injuries. The result, it is hoped, will be a paradigm shift toward quicker solutions to the gaps in any one of the isolated specialties. "It is an exciting era of hearing research," he wrote.

• • •

Big pharma may not yet be involved in finding a prevention or cure for hearing loss, but small biotech is on the case. Jonathan Kil, who formerly worked in Ed Rubel's lab at UW, is the president and CEO of Sound Pharmaceuticals, a small company in Seattle. Kil is trying to develop a prophylactic to help prevent hearing loss.

The compound he is working with is a synthetic antioxidant called ebselen. Kil tried for some years to interest the military in developing it, but is now focusing on civilians, especially teenagers.

A 2011 article on *Xconomy*, a webzine with a Seattle focus, quoted him as saying that the military was stretched too thin to provide volunteers. Kil says they turned their attention instead to the Hearing Pill marketed by American BioHealth.

Ebselen is recognized as effective in the early treatment of a stroke. Ebselen (SPI-1005), the Sound Pharmaceuticals compound, is designed to mimic an enzyme in the inner ear that decreases when the ear is exposed to loud noise.

In 2012, when I met with Kil at his lab, he and his colleague Eric D. Lynch were in Phase 2 FDA trials for the compound used as a prophylactic against hearing loss. Colleen Le Prell at the University of Florida was to conduct the clinical trial. Her team would recruit eighty young people as subjects, randomly assigned to a placebo or a low, medium, or high dose of ebselen. The drug (or placebo) would be given for two days before exposure to four hours of loud music, through an iPod, loud enough to cause a temporary threshold shift and for two days after. The subjects would be studied fourteen days after exposure, to see the level of damage remaining to the hair cells. (Given what we now know from the work of Sharon Kujawa and Charles Liberman about the long-term damage from temporary threshold shift, this seems possibly risky to the subjects.)

Kil is planning another SPI-1005 clinical trial, for which they will restrict the enrollment to those with slight hearing loss, but they are not now planning to test ebselen for chronic conditions like age-related hearing loss. "If everything falls into place, we could file an NDA [New Drug Application] at the end of 2014–2015," he told me.

Despite my asking four or five times during our interview, and again in a follow-up e-mail, how ebselen would be administered once it got FDA approval, Kil never answered the question. Would it be administered like a daily vitamin? I asked repeatedly. The clinical trials so far test the effectiveness only against a onetime planned exposure. But teenagers listen to their iPods continuously, as any parent knows. A simpler solution is to get teenagers to turn down the volume.

Sound Pharmaceuticals has a second drug in Phase 2 trials, an ebselen-allopurinol combination which might be used to protect against chemotherapeutic exposure to ototoxins.

Kil and his former mentor Ed Rubel have exchanged some sharp words over the Internet, and it's difficult for a layperson to weigh in on the dispute. Suffice it to say that Rubel acknowledges that ebselen works to some degree—like any antioxidant ("you can do it with strawberries")—in that it tips the cell away from dying, but just a bit. "I don't have any doubt that ebselen works. On a very small part of the dose-response curve. But a drug company isn't going to do anything that is a small part of the dose-response curve." His online comments were less modulated.

For his part, Kil responds that the ivory tower is not a place to develop real-world drugs. "I understand that academics can make nice discoveries, but getting a product approved, the academic doesn't want to go beyond target identification and validation. And just the budget it takes to get through preclinical testing of a new drug product can be . . . the NIH isn't really set up to fund that."

Rubel disagrees. He points out that his and other labs are doing just that through the NIH Blueprint Neurotherapeutics Network initiative.

• • •

Robert Jackler at Stanford would also disagree. I suspect he spoke for many academic researchers in his vision of the university's role in the search for a cure for hearing loss. In his enthusiasm for the scope of the effort, he invoked the moon shot; the search for a cure for cancer, for polio, for smallpox; the development of the atom bomb—all in the space of a few sentences.

But his enthusiasm seems well-founded. "The thing about this program here is that Stanford is a very collaborative, collegial, and interdisciplinary place," he said. "It's a place where I can go out and successfully recruit the very best people. And by having a group of really incredibly creative good people, you're able to bring them together into a critical mass, almost like a Los Alamos concept, right? You bring the best and brightest together, you provide them the resources, and they're all driven toward this. There's a clear goal. We're all working on regenerating that hair cell, coming from many different approaches. We're working with geneticists, molecular biologists, developmental biologists. And engineers to help with the delivery.

"When you define a great vision—'We want to cure hearing loss'—you get a lot of people very excited about it," he went on. But he calls it "realistic optimism," understanding that it takes "sustained effort over a long period of time. And the resources to lubricate that effort."

The resources in this case include not only the seventy scientists at Stanford working on hearing regeneration, but money. Stanford has a fund-raising goal for hearing research over the next ten years of $170 million. Jackler has every hope of achieving that goal: "How often can you say, 'We might categorically overcome a major type of human suffering'?"

With such a large and concentrated group of scientists, Stanford is able to think about the problem in a variety of ways, using different strategies. "You start off with six or eight different strategies. You put early-stage efforts into them, and then over time you concentrate." The cochlear implant, he went on, offers the "miracle of partially replacing a lost sense in humans for the very first time." But, he said, the implant is limited: it's not perfect in sound reproduction, it's extraordinarily expensive, and it's not applicable to the millions and millions of hard of hearing who are not deaf.

Nor is it available to the majority of people with severe hearing loss around the world. Jackler believes a biological cure would be. "We hope that it is made so simple that it could be an eardrop. Will it be something that a barefoot doctor in western China could do? Perhaps not."

But on the other hand, he muses, perhaps it will be. If a pharmaceutical company eventually brought it along through the regulatory channels and clinical trials, that company might someday be able to recoup their huge investment. Once they recoup the investment, once they can produce it "in fifty-five-gallon drums," Jackler said, they can make it available to the millions who need it.

"The analogy is perhaps HIV drugs," he said. "We would very much like to be able to see this as something that could universally help people, not just in wealthy, technologically advanced societies."

• • •

Jackler is a strong and articulate voice for hair cell regeneration research, and his department is impressive, and growing. The University of Washington has had its own hair cell regeneration initiative since 2000, with a multi-investigator team for over fifteen years. Much of the early research was done there, and much important work continues. Not lightly did George Gates refer to Rubel as the godfather of hair cell regeneration.

Today, with the backing of the Hearing Health Foundation and its consortium of members sharing research and findings, the field is stronger than ever—with scientists from institutions all over the country working collaboratively. The excitement among researchers is palpable, and the advances after many years of hard work are finally producing significant results. For those millions of people with hearing loss, the prospect of a biological cure is at last a reality. A distant reality, perhaps, but no less dazzling for it.

VOICES: EUGENE KAPLAN

At least a dozen psychoanalysts answered a query posted by Leon Hoffman, president of the American Psychoanalytic Association, on the group's website, saying a writer was looking for late-deafened therapists for a book project. Eugene Kaplan was not one of them, but several analysts who did respond suggested that I talk to him. I tracked him down at the University of South Carolina School of Medicine.

Kaplan, a professor at several notable New York medical schools before moving to South Carolina in 1985, answered me promptly, and we fell into an e-mail discussion about his hearing loss, my hearing loss, and how people in general deal with it. Being a psychoanalyst, he was particularly interested in the psychological ramifications of midlife hearing loss. But he also talked about his own loss, often poignantly, in a formal tone that reminded me of Isaiah Jackson's.

"I started losing my hearing in my late forties," he wrote to me. The cause was unknown. "Too much time had elapsed since WWII combat for it to be trauma-related. Then an older cousin reminded me that our grandmother was deaf, and that she herself had significant hearing loss. Fancy name: familial early-onset neurosensory deafness."

Like most of us, he refused to acknowledge the problem at first. "My denial was shattered when a patient informed me that I had misheard the word upon which my brilliant interpretation of her dream was based. (Dreams present us with difficulties similar to names and numbers: no logical context.)" Since this was an e-mail, I couldn't hear his voice, but I suspected he was smiling wryly as he wrote this.

He chose not to make his hearing loss visible. "My response," he wrote, "bilateral aids concealed in my glasses; it took some years to overcome my self-consciousness." He made the kind of arrangements that maximized his ability to hear: moving out of an office with a noisy window air conditioner into one centrally air-conditioned and, as he said, "a repositioning of the couch so I could see the patient's lips."

He was a skilled lip-reader. "Prior to my cochlear implant over five years ago, lipreading raised my comprehension from fifteen to seventy-five percent."

One of the more common responses to deafness was not an option for him: faking it. "In practice, I simply could not afford to smile and pretend that I understood, so I asked again. After the second time, I'd asked for spelling or even a written clarification. My unapologetic motto: Better an analyst who cannot hear than one who does not listen!"

Kaplan is now eighty-five. "Having lived with progressive deafness almost forty years," he wrote, "I know when to stop butting against the brick wall, and to look for ways around it. I've been most fortunate to have control of the treatment setting to maximize the intelligibility of speech, by keeping background noise to a minimum and only one of us talking at a time.

"When I left private practice in Great Neck in 1985 for a professorship at our medical school here," he went on, "I applied the same principles: I chair, Robert's Rules, one speaker at a time." For people with hearing loss, that one speaker can too often be themselves (it's so much easier than trying to hear the others). "Hard-of-hearing people have a well-deserved reputation for garrulousness. Easy to understand: as long as they're talking, they know what's being said.

"I eventually became resigned to missing out on the cocktail and dinner party conversations," he wrote. "I never overcame the irretrievable loss of conversations with my grandkids when they were still little and their pronunciation was hard to follow.

"This should provide some grist for your mill," he ended. I hope someday to meet him.

Epilogue: In the Land of the Near Deaf

Despite advances in technology, and despite the promise of a cure, hearing loss is permanent, at least for now. Once you enter the land of the near deaf, you don't leave.

But you can learn to make it feel like home. As I've come to accept my hearing loss, I've replaced denial and anger with something more productive. I know I have to work to hear, that I have to practice hearing and I have to practice listening. I have to turn off the captions on the TV. I have to listen to recorded books. I have to pay attention and force my brain to work as hard as it can to understand, instead of shrugging and giving up.

With my hearing aid and cochlear implant, and with practice, I can hear much that I couldn't as recently as two years ago. I can hear birds. I can hear a rushing stream. I can hear a car coming up behind me on a country road. I can hear the funny half growl, half whimper my dog makes when he wants to go out. I can catch snippets of overheard conversations. I'm beginning to go to the movies again.

One thing I probably won't be able to hear is music. I can hear a solo voice. I can sometimes hear a solo instrument. But I'll never again hear Bruce Springsteen, U2, the Rolling Stones, Eric Clapton and B.B. King, Paul Simon—the noise of the multiple instruments eclipses the sound of the voice. I can't hear harmony. I can't hear an orchestra. I'll never again hear a Mahler symphony or a Mozart opera, Verdi, Wagner, church music, a children's choir. Unheard melodies are not sweeter. The joy of a truly glorious piece of music, the emotional depths it can stir, are gone for me, unlikely to be restored.

• • •

Despite the imperfection of hearing instruments, it's a good time to be deaf. Hearing aids and cochlear implants are increasingly sophisticated, and someday soon will come close to mimicking the human ear.

Hearing aids are widely available, and are sometimes even reasonable in cost. Cochlear implants are more and more often an option for people with hearing loss, and insurance will pay for them. When Dr. Hoffman first talked to me about a cochlear implant, five or six years ago, despite poor hearing in my right ear and profound deafness in my left, I would not have met FDA standards. Today I would (and did). Assistive listening devices like FM systems and hearing loops mean that people with serious hearing loss can hear in places they'd never have been able to previously—in noisy crowded public spaces, at the theater and movies, at parties, in churches.

Critics like Sherry Turkle, author of *Alone Together: Why We Expect More from Technology and Less from Each Other*, bemoan the death of conversation, the isolation of communicating through e-mail or text. But for those with hearing loss—and many others who for one reason or another are not able to easily converse—e-mail and texting are the lifelines that allow us to continue to be part of the world.

• • •

I spent much of my adult life—both personal and professional—faking it. Not even my closest friends knew the extent of my hearing loss. For those who have hearing loss, I hope that, like me, they'll eventually discover the immense relief, the freedom of coming clean. And by describing the daily obstacles that a hearing-impaired person faces, I hope that those who live with—or work with or love or teach or minister to—someone with a hearing impairment will better understand their experience, the hard work, the emotional upheaval, the anger and pain.

The more I learned about hearing impairment—and the more I talked to people with hearing loss—the more I realized that most people suffer their loss in isolation, as I did. Most don't know others like them. They don't understand that they have millions of unhappy compatriots. Hearing loss remains a silent and invisible disability. It needn't be. There are lots of us out there.

For decades I pretended to be "normal." I didn't subscribe to hearing loss magazines or make any effort to find others like me. The books I read were about the Deaf—not me. When I got a cochlear implant, the books I read were about the miracle of regaining your hearing. I'm writing this book for people like me—not Deaf, not miraculously cured.

Despite my sophisticated devices, I still can't hear well enough to follow a conversation except under optimum circumstances—one-on-one, facing each other, in a quiet place. I hear speech, but I often don't understand it. I hear the beginning and end of sentences, I catch stray words, I can occasionally tell if someone has an accent. Like David Lodge nuzzling the bosom of the lady in the red dress, I tilt and bend and shift position, twisting myself in knots, to maximize my hearing.

And, alas, even though I'm open about my hearing loss, I still guess at what's been said, and often get it wrong.

"When are we eating?" my husband says.

"Chicken," I answer.

Notes

Introduction

Perhaps the biggest problem in writing about hearing loss is determining how many people it affects, and how. All the notes in the Introduction (with the exception of the last) are about statistics.

For instance, in the United States, where we are good at counting things, I found a range of statistics for something as simple as how many are affected by hearing loss. The National Institute on Deafness and Other Communication Disorders sets the number at 36 million, while other organizations offer higher or lower figures. Part of the NIH, the NIDCD seemed like an impeccable source. So I went with their number. Then, in November 2011, Johns Hopkins researcher Frank R. Lin and his colleagues published a credible epidemiological study that blew the NIDCD figure out of the water. Lin found that 48 million Americans suffer hearing impairment ("Hearing Loss Prevalence in the United States," by Frank R. Lin, John K. Niparko, and Luigi Ferrucci, *Archives of Internal Medicine*, November 14, 2011). How could these two disparate figures both be right? An NIDCD official explained that the NIDCD numbers were "reported" hearing loss—that is, people who had self-identified as having hearing loss. Frank Lin's numbers were derived from audiometric testing. The Lin database was the National Health and Nutrition Examination Survey (NHANES), a long-term statistical database, which reflects hearing test results rather than self-reporting. I have used his figures. The figure for the percentage of Americans with hearing loss under the age of sixty (55 percent) is from "The Impact of Treated Hearing Loss on Quality of Life," Sergei Kochkin, Better Hearing Institute.

The *JAMA* study "Change in Prevalence of Hearing Loss in US Adolescents," by Josef Shargorodsky, Sharon G. Curhan, Gary C. Curhan, and Roland Eavey, August 18, 2010, will be discussed at greater length in the notes for chapter 3.

There is no question that the elderly account for a majority of those with hearing loss. But determining a demographic breakdown of those statistics, even in the United States, is also difficult. Frank Lin and his colleagues state that "two-thirds of Americans seventy and over are hearing impaired" ("Hearing Loss Prevalence and Risk Factors Among Older Adults in the United States," by Frank R. Lin,

Roland Thorpe, Sandra Gordon-Salant, and Luigi Ferrucci, *Journal of Gerontology*, May 2011). The NIDCD reports that "forty-seven percent of adults seventy-five years old or older have a hearing impairment" (NIDCD Quick Statistics). Many factors explain why these two figures, which should be comparable, are in fact as different as apples and oranges. How is "hearing impaired" defined? How is the number determined (audiometric testing or self-report)? Who is included in the count? (The CDC, for instance, counts only non-institutionalized adults.) Lin's figure is for those over seventy, the NIDCD's for those over seventy-five. Finally, and significantly, any statistics derived from self-reporting must take into account the fact that a large proportion of those with hearing loss deny it to themselves and to others. As for the comment "But in only 8 percent of men and 16 percent of women did the loss begin after the age of seventy," the source is the NIDCD graphic "Age at Which Hearing Loss Begins."

Determining how many people worldwide suffer hearing loss is even more difficult than counting domestically. WHO updated its 2000 report on "The Global Burden of Hearing Loss" in March of 2012, and gave an overall figure of 275 million. *Hearing International,* an online magazine about global hearing issues, cites a worldwide figure of 250 million with *moderate or worse* hearing loss, and 600 million overall. Hear-it, a noncommercial website published in Belgium, cites Professor Adrian Davis of the British MRC Institute of Hearing Research, who estimates that the total number of people suffering from hearing loss of more than 25 dB's will exceed 700 million by 2015. Hear-it also estimated numbers for individual regions and countries to the best of its ability. In some cases the information is vague indeed: "Asia is the most densely populated continent and most likely the one with the greatest number of hearing impaired people." For Africa, the report states: "It is difficult to get a precise picture of the prevalence and causes of hearing loss in Africa."

The same kinds of problems are encountered with measuring the use of hearing aids. The NIDCD says only one in five who would benefit uses a hearing aid. Frank Lin and Wade Chien say one in seven: "Prevalence of Hearing Aid Use Among Older Adults in the United States, *Archives of Internal Medicine,* February 13, 2012. By either count, there are a lot of people with uncorrected hearing loss. An ongoing MarkeTrak study, published since 2004 under the aegis of the Better Hearing Institute, and based on self-reporting in more than eighty thousand households, tracks trends in the hearing health market and is an excellent source for detailed demographic information. MarkeTrak VIII, published in November 2009, appeared in *Hearing Review.* Sergei Kochkin is executive director of the Better Hearing Institute, and the author of the report.

1. Losing It

Jess Dancer's observations about the bimodal nature of hearing (*Advance for Hearing Practice Management,* May 27, 2008) are something that every person with hearing loss intuitively understands. If I watch a TV show with simultaneous captions, I can hear and understand the words the actors are saying. Without captions I can only hear that they are saying *something,* but I can't identify what.

Tina Lannin's lip-read report of what was said by the participants at the royal wedding was reprinted in www.hearinglossweb.com in May 2011. Hearinglossweb is a compendium of news and information of interest to those with adult-onset hearing loss. The editors are Char and Larry Sivertson, who both suffered hearing loss as adults. Their newsletter is weekly and is impressively organized, so that a reader may, for instance, easily find many articles on hearing loss in the military, in a single file, footnoted with the original documentation.

Much of the information on speechreading comes from Mark Ross, Ph.D., professor emeritus of Audiology at the University of Connecticut. He is a longtime columnist for *Hearing Loss* magazine. This article appeared on the website www.therubins .com.

When I began to wonder about the voices I hear in dreams, I naturally turned to Freud. Mikko Keskinen's "Hearing Voices in Dreams: Freud's Tossing and Turning with Speech and Writing" appeared in an online journal for the psychological study of the arts, *PsyART*, May 29, 2002.

I have quoted in several places from George Prochnik's 2010 book *In Pursuit of Silence*, which I also reviewed for *The New York Times*. Prochnik's narrative is a totally enjoyable journey in search of perfect quiet. Along the way he also encounters the loudest noises he can find.

In the spring of 2011, I spent several days at Johns Hopkins. The information from Brad May is from one of the interviews I did there. Johns Hopkins has a major clinical and research otolaryngology department, and many of the researchers are also clinicians. Hopkins is one of the major centers for cochlear implants.

This quote from Stefan Heller appeared in the *Journal of Communication Disorders* in 2010. I visited him at Stanford in 2012, where he is working on a biological cure for hearing loss. That material appears in chapter 12.

For years it never occurred to me that I would have trouble hearing a fire alarm. But late in 2012, I happened to hear Laura Squassoni of the New York Fire Department speak to the Manhattan Chapter of the HLAA about fire safety for the hard of hearing. As part of an FDNY grant, she was able to give each of us a Lifetone HL bedside fire alarm, which works with a standard smoke alarm to alert those who might not hear the high-frequency pitch of the ordinary smoke alarm. The Lifetone (available on Amazon.com) picks up the pattern of signals from the regular detector and emits its own low-frequency alarm, which is more likely to be audible to people with hearing loss. The Lifetone includes a "bed shaker" that can be put under the pillow or the mattress. I was flabbergasted that in all my research—at the HLAA meetings I've attended, at scores of visits to audiologists—I had never heard of this kind of alarm, a potentially literally lifesaving device for the hard of hearing.

2. Why?

Statistics, again, are hard to pin down. The figures for the percentage of Americans who develop hearing loss during certain decades of their lives come from the NIDCD. That study does not specify prevalence in people in their eighties, however. Those figures (for people eighty and over) come from a study published in May 2011, "The Prevalence of Hearing Impairment and Associated Risk Factors," by Scott D. Nash et al., *Archives of Otolaryngology–Head and Neck Surgery*. Nash's database was the Epidemiology of Hearing Loss Study, an ongoing population-based cohort study begun in 1993 in Beaver Dam, Wisconsin. The Nash study gives an overall figure for U.S. hearing loss as 29 million, much lower than Frank Lin's 48 million and even than the NIDCD's 36 million.

The link between hearing loss and cardiovascular disease is discussed in an article by George A. Gates et al. in the *Archives of Otolaryngology–Head and Neck Surgery*, February 1993. Gates observed: "There is a small but statistically significant association of cardiovascular disease and hearing status in the elderly that is greater for women than men and more in the low than the high frequencies." The study noted that the low-frequency loss that typically comes with presbycusis, or age-related hearing loss, is classically associated with microvascular disease leading to atrophy of the striavascularis (part of the auditory nerve). The long-term Framingham Heart Study also found a link between low-frequency hearing loss and a variety of cardiovascular events.

I had a great deal of help with the wording on decibel levels from the composer and former record producer Richard Einhorn and from Brad Ingrao, a well-known audiologist.

Sharon Kujawa and Charles Liberman's study on the long-term damage from early exposure to moderate levels of noise offers an interesting and potentially significant perspective on noise and age-related hearing loss. Their paper "Adding Insult to Injury: Cochlear Nerve Degeneration After 'Temporary' Noise-Induced Hearing Loss" appeared in the *Journal of Neuroscience*, November 11, 2009. Kujawa also discussed the implications of the finding at the 2011 Research Symposium at the HLAA annual conference. Liberman discussed it further in an interview in Cambridge in 2012. (Kujawa was out of town.)

I owe much of my information on the workings of the inner ear to Brad May, of Hopkins, who patiently walked me through elementary otolaryngology in a 2011 interview. He also explained why it is that people with mild to moderate hearing loss can hear a voice clearly but not understand what is said.

Sharon Kujawa's talk at HLAA was also very helpful in deciphering the structure of the inner ear and what can go wrong. The reference to the long-term fate of SGCs is from the paper previously noted, "Adding Insult to Injury . . ."

The material about noise exposure in infants, especially white noise, and its potential long-term effects came primarily from Brad May. The material seems obscure—even some otolaryngologists I talked to weren't sure what the medial olivocochlear system was—but knowledge of it could protect some vulnerable infants from later hearing and perceptual difficulties. A. M. Lauer and Brad May discussed the MOC system and their research in "The Medial Olivocochlear System Attenuates the Developmental Impact of Early Noise Exposure," published in *JARO, Journal of the Association for Research in Otolaryngology*, 2011.

Frank Lin et al. wrote about the racial disparity in rates of hearing loss in the previously cited "Hearing Loss Prevalence and Risk Factors Among Older Adults in the United States," in the *Journal of Gerontology* in 2011. We also discussed his thoughts about the role of melanin in an interview at Hopkins in 2011. I'm not aware of studies following up on the suggestion that melanin might be adapted as a preventive for hearing loss.

The cause of sudden hearing loss is known in only 10 to 15 percent of cases. This figure comes from an NIDCD online posting on sudden deafness. Other sources phrase the cause as "seventy-five percent unknown."

3. Bring in 'Da Noise!

Sepp Blatter's comment about Africa having "a different rhythm, a different sound" appeared originally in a blog post and was picked up by many in the news media. The decibel levels were reported differently in different media, but by any measure they were very loud.

The competition for the loudest football stadium yielded many amusing and alarming facts. The sources are noted in the text. In some cases they are established news organizations like ESPN or *Sports Illustrated*. In others they are sports blogs.

Alan Schwarz's *New York Times* article appeared on June 6, 2011, under the headline "Stoking Excitement, Arenas Pump Up the Volume."

Haile Gebrselassie's musical preferences were reported in *The New York Times* on January 10, 2008. "They're Playing My Song. Time to Work Out." The article also reported on Costas Karageorghis's suggested workout playlists.

The negative comment about The Who's performance at Super Bowl XLIV came from a blogger who called himself (or herself) Who-Fan, in a comment on *Rolling Stone*'s website.

The competition for loudest band is one carried on informally online. Many of the measurements are not official.

The description of the premiere performance of Mahler's Eighth Symphony can be found online in *The Flying Inkpot* # 74, the Classical Music Reviews, by Derek Lim. Gustavo Dudamel's performance with 1400 musicians was reported on his website. The concert was broadcast on *LA Phil Live*.

The *Times* article was headlined: "At Home With: Ved Mehta; In a Dark Harbor, a Bright House," by John Leland, May 22, 2003.

The fact that loud music speeds up the rate of drinking comes from "Why Loud Music in Bars Increases Alcohol Consumption," by Nicolas Guéguen et al., *Alcoholism: Clinical & Experimental Research*, July 21, 2001.

Celebrity chefs and their musical preferences have been reported in various media outlets.

The researchers Tara P. McAlexander, Richard Neitzel, and Robyn R. M. Gershon conducted the study of New York's public spaces. The research was sponsored by the University of Washington School of Public Health and the Mailman School of Public Health at Columbia University, which published a pilot study in 2010 on the New York City Urban Soundscape. The study on New York's mass transit system appeared in the *American Journal of Public Health*, August 2009.

George Prochnik was the first to make me aware of J. M. Picker's "The Sound-proof Study: Victorian Professionals, Work Space and Urban Noise," published in *Victorian Soundscapes* and available online. Most of the material about Dickens's London comes from this work, except where noted otherwise. It is Prochnik who wrote of Carlyle's study that it had somehow ended up being the noisiest room in the house.

David Nasaw's *Children of the City: At Work and at Play*, Anchor Press/ Doubleday, 1985, looks at New York in the same period.

The conflicting studies that have come out recently on the issue of teenage hearing health are a dazzling example of how statistics get manipulated, and how the same numbers can lead to completely opposite conclusions. The following paragraphs discuss this in more detail. It's important to understand why the information on hearing loss in teenagers seems so conflicted.

Two articles published within months of each other in August 2010 and winter of 2010–2011 created the controversy over an increase in teenage hearing loss. Both were published by Harvard-affiliated groups: Dr. Josef Shargorodsky and his colleagues at the Channing Laboratory at Brigham and Women's Hospital in Cambridge published the first, and a few months later Elisabeth Henderson and others at the Massachusetts Eye and Ear Infirmary (Henderson, with a B.A., was a student at Harvard Medical School) published the second. Both studies relied on the same database: the National Health and Nutrition Examination Survey (NHANES), which compared hearing levels of children between 1988 and 1994, and hearing levels in the same age group in 2005–2006.

Shargorodsky's study was published in the *Journal of the American Medical Association* under the neutral title "Change in Prevalence of Hearing Loss in US Adolescents." The paper noted that the earlier NHANES study had found high- or low-frequency hearing loss in at least one ear in 14.9 percent of children aged six to nineteen, and 12.9 percent had audiometric evidence of noise-induced hearing loss. For their study, the Shargorodsky group did some complicated statistical adjustment that allowed them to focus on twelve-to-nineteen-year-olds. They found that "the prevalence of any hearing loss increased significantly from 14.9 percent . . . to 19.5 percent." The "results" section, from which this quote comes, also noted that the hearing loss was more commonly unilateral and involved the high frequencies. Teenagers from low-income households had "significantly higher odds of hearing loss."

The reputable American Speech-Language-Hearing Association headlined its online report in *The ASHA Leader*: "Teens at Risk: 'We're on the Edge of an Epidemic.'" Citing the 14.9 to 19.5 increase, the many media reports that followed almost universally used the term "epidemic" and translated the statistics as "an increase of thirty-one percent." Most failed to mention that it was unilateral.

Three months later, Elisabeth Henderson and her group (which included a Ph.D. and an M.D.) came out with a study titled "Prevalence of Noise-Induced Hearing-Threshold Shift and Hearing Loss Among U.S. Youths" in *Pediatrics*. (Hearing threshold, as discussed earlier, is the quietest sound a person can hear. Threshold shift usually suggests that the threshold has been raised and the person is hearing less well than they did before.) Henderson et al. studied the results from the same adolescents twelve to nineteen years old, although for some reason Henderson's total number came to only 4310 instead of the 4699 that the Shargorodsky group studied. Though Henderson et al. also studied high- and low-frequency readings, they used a different measure called "noise-induced threshold shift," or NITS. They found "no significant increases" between study periods. They did find a small increase among females, where the NITS went from 11.6 percent to 16.7 percent between the two survey periods. Most comments skipped over this fact. The use of noise protection devices was lower among females.

Like the Shargorodsky study, this one found a greater incidence of hearing loss among low-income teenagers. Though the Henderson study found no increase in hearing loss (except among those girls), it did find a huge increase in exposure to noise, perhaps the most significant finding. "The overall prevalence of exposure to loud noise or listening to music through headphones in the previous 24 hours increased from 19.8% to 34%."

At the Hearing Loss Association of America's annual meeting in Washington, D.C., in June 2011, Dr. William Clark, director of the Program of Audiology and Communication Sciences at Washington University School of Medicine, discussed these two studies at length. He focused not only on misuse of statistics but also on the frequently overlooked fact that in the majority of the cases where there was hearing loss, the loss was in one ear. As he logically pointed out, there are "several factors that are inconsistent with noise exposure here," including the fact that a large number of the cases were unilateral. Most people, as he pointed out, listen to their MP3 players with both ears.

He then offered some surprising findings by comparing an even earlier NHANES study done in 1966 to 1970. He found that the left ear data for boys twelve to nineteen, where most of the hearing loss occurred, remained unchanged from 1966 to 1970. "Actually, kids hear better today than they did in 1966–1970." And probably better than they ever have because they are generally healthier than they've ever been. "I found some old data back to the 1940s which suggested that hearing just continued to get better in kids," Dr. Clark went on. "I think that's really not surprising if you think about the fact that kids are healthier, they have better nutrition. If you look at state high school athletic records, they're all better now than they were in 1990 and 1980. They have better hearing in this case."

Still, he hastened to emphasize that the threat to adolescents' hearing remains very real: "Remember that iPods and personal listening devices are very, very common these days, usage has greatly increased, and as Dr. Kujawa [the previous speaker] mentioned, the hazard that is posed by these devices—and by any noise exposure—is a combination of how loud it is and how long you listen to it."

4. You Can't See It, but I Can't Hear You

"Hearing Loss and Incident Dementia" by Frank R. Lin, Jeffrey Metter, Richard J. O'Brien, Susan M. Resnick, Alan B. Zonderman, and Luigi Ferrucci, *Archives of Neurology*, February 2011, is fascinating, and for someone with impaired hearing, alarming. The participants underwent audiometric testing when they entered the study, between 1990 and 1994. All were dementia free. The median follow-up period was 11.9 years, with some participants studied for as long as 18 years. Although the study found that hearing loss is independently associated with incident "all-cause" dementia, it did not ascertain whether it was a marker for early stage dementia or "a modifiable risk factor for dementia."

What the Lin study did not address was how often hearing loss may be mistaken for dementia. An elderly person is taken to the emergency room and only after the family arrives some time later does anyone say, "Where are Mom's hearing aids?" Meanwhile, the staff, unable to communicate with her, has noted "dementia" on the chart.

Gallaudet University has published a time line of events in Deaf culture, collated by Wendy Shaner. The first item on Shaner's time line is 1000 B.C., "Hebrew Law Denies Deaf Rights." Info.com, which has also published a deaf time line, goes on to discuss Plato, Aristotle, and Saint Augustine's views of deafness. Because many "deaf" people have some degree of hearing—correctable to some extent with hearing aids or even an ear trumpet—"deafness" in these passages refers also to what we would call "hard of hearing."

Regi Theodor Enerstvedt's *Legacy of the Past* devotes one of its three chapters to "The Development of Education for Deaf People." It is available online.

Todd Bentley's *The Revelation of the Deaf and Dumb Spirit* is an online publication, found on a website called GodSpeak International. As noted, he has been evicted from his own church. Todd Bentley's observation about mental and physical impairment in the deaf has some basis in fact. Deafness may be a symptom of a syndromic disorder with other physical and mental symptoms. But the far larger majority of the deaf are otherwise perfectly healthy. Before the deaf were given access to education and taught to speak, they did seem "deaf and dumb," but that has not been the case for two hundred years.

Mark Ross, who also provided much of the information on speechreading in chapter 1, is an audiologist and longtime contributor to *Hearing Loss,* the journal of the HLAA. This article appeared in *Hearing Loss*, in the May/June 2010 issue.

David Lodge discussed his hearing loss with Moira Petty in the *Mail Online*: "How Hiding His Deafness Ruined Novelist David's Lodge's Life," May 20, 2008. I didn't know that Lodge had hearing loss when I read *Deaf Sentence* (Viking, 2008), but his description of unacknowledged hearing impairment is so hilariously and cringingly familiar that I was sure he must be. Lodge told the interviewer that he had tried to hide his deafness for ten years.

Evelyn Waugh and Harriet Martineau are both quoted in the excellent compendium of references to deafness, *The Quiet Ear: Deafness in Literature*, edited by Brian Grant, Faber and Faber, 1988.

D. D. Guttenplan mentions I.F. Stone's hearing loss in his 2009 biography, *American Radical: The Life and Times of I.F. Stone*. This quote comes from a commentary that appeared in the Muskegon *Opinion*.

Megan McKinney's *The Magnificent Medills* was published in 2011, by Harper-Collins. This quote appears on page 32.

The anecdote about Ian Waterman, who had lost all sense of touch, including the feeling of his feet on the floor, is described in "The Importance of the Sense of Touch in Virtual and Real Environments," by G. Robles-De-La-Torre, published by the International Society for Haptics. Haptics is the study of touch in real and virtual environments.

Chef Grant Achatz was the subject of an interview with NPR, "The Chef Who Lost His Sense of Taste," at the time of the publication of his book *Life, on the Line: A Chef's Story of Chasing Greatness, Facing Death, and Redefining the Way We Eat*, Gotham, 2011.

Robin Marantz Henig is a friend and fellow science writer. She wrote about the loss of her sense of smell after a fall in "Something's Off," *The New York Times Magazine*, October 17, 2004. I would often go for walks in the park with her at that time, and I remember standing next to a blossoming apple tree, describing the smell to her—sweet and slightly spicy. By hearing these descriptions, she began to train her brain to remember the smells. In the same way, as I tried to regain my hearing after I got a cochlear implant, Cory Dean, another friend, would describe noises for me. Once, walking under a tree full of twittering birds, she asked if I heard them. I had heard something but I didn't know what it was. When she pointed out the tree with the birds, the undefined noise became recognizable as birds.

Jack Ashley's remarks are quoted in *The Quiet Ear*, page 47.

Mary Kaland and Kate Salvatore's article "The Psychology of Hearing Loss" was published in *The ASHA Leader* (the publication of the American Speech-Language-Hearing Association), March 19, 2002.

The filmmaker Maryte Kavaliauskas talked about David Hockney's work in an interview with PBS's *American Masters*, which aired her film. Trip Gabriel's "At Home With/David Hockney; Acquainted With the Light" appeared in *The New York Times* on January 21, 1993.

5. Am I Deaf or Just Dumb?

The findings about psychological "disturbances" being fourfold greater among people with hearing loss are cited in "Auditory Physiology and Perception," by Bradford J. May and John K. Niparko, chapter 1 in Niparko: *Cochlear Implants: Principles and Practices*, 2nd edition, Lippincott Williams & Wilkins, 2009. May and Niparko cite a 1990 study, "Quality-of-Life Changes and Hearing Impairment. A Randomized Trial," by C. D. Mulrow et al., *Annals of Internal Medicine*, 1990.

Norman Doidge's *The Brain That Changes Itself* was published in 2007 by Viking Press. This quote appears on page 68 in a chapter about Michael Merzenich, emeritus professor in neuroscience at the University of California, San Francisco, and one of the world's leading researchers on brain plasticity. He led the cochlear implant team at UCSF, which transferred its technology to Advanced Bionics, makers of my implant. One of the most difficult things to remember is a person's name. The signal, as Doidge refers to it, is rarely clear: a name has no clues unless it's accompanied by contextual information, such as: "Do you know Professor So-and-So, whose book *This and That* has been receiving such great reviews?" "I'm So-and-So, Katie's older sister from Seattle." Worst are people who simply say, "Hi, I'm Bruce." Uh, hi.

These lines from Beethoven are contained in the Heiligenstadt Testament, dated October 6, 1802. "With joy I hasten toward death," the thirty-two-year-old Beethoven wrote. He died in 1827.

Hear Again, a collection of e-mails that Arlene Romoff wrote to family and friends as she was going through the process of a cochlear implant, was published in 1999 by the League for the Hard of Hearing. Romoff also wrote about getting a second implant in *Listening Closely: A Journey to Bilateral Hearing*, Imagine, 2011.

Richard Reed gave a workshop at the 2011 HLAA conference in Washington. He's a witty speaker and the room was packed. Describing what he heard after he got his implant, he said, "Family and friends sounded like giant chipmunks. I heard percussive noises everywhere: the sound of walking, my corduroys rubbing." At the end of the talk, he played a composition based on "Twinkle Twinkle Little Star," which, as he pointed out, contains some dark moments in the rarely sung later verses. "Twinkle

Twinkle" was the first music he recognized after his implant, and this is a bluesy jazz variation that brings out those somber undertones.

The relationship between hearing loss and cardiovascular events is an association, not a cause and effect. Friedland's study, presented at an otolaryngology conference, was the subject of an article he wrote for *ENT Today*, September 2009.

6. "They Don't Scream, 'I'M WEARING HEARING AIDS!!!'"

Sergei Kochkin's comments on the Lin study appeared as an online comment in an article in *Hearing News Watch* about the Lin study. As noted earlier, he is executive director of the Better Hearing Institute, which conducts and publishes the MarkeTrak studies.

My insurance company reimbursed me $500 of the $6000 I spent for my first two hearing aids, in 2002. My current insurance company gives no reimbursement for hearing aids; Medicare does not cover hearing exams or hearing aids except in special circumstances. Medicaid policies differ from state to state. For a list of services state by state, go to www.hearingloss.org/content/medicaid-regulations.

The figures for hearing aid use by men as opposed to women are also disputed. The NIDCD reported that the rate of hearing aid use for adults with moderate to severe hearing loss was 194.8 per thousand for females and 132.2 for males (in 2001). The MarkeTrak studies find greater use by males.

The kidnapped British woman, Judith Tebbutt, was released in return for a $1 million ransom, paid by friends, in March 2012. The reference to her severe hearing impairment was in *The New York Times*, September 12, 2011. Some newspapers reported that she wore a hearing aid or hearing "aids."

John Tierney's article was at the top of the most e-mailed list for several days straight. It generated hope and excitement among people with hearing loss, and many friends asked me if I was going to install a loop system at home. It *is* possible to loop a room in your home—or many rooms—but it's relatively expensive and the looping only works when you're in that room. David Myers, a social psychologist at Hope College, gave the keynote address at the 2012 HLAA convention. He is an advocate for looping, and has been in the forefront of getting public spaces like houses of worship and airports to install looping systems. John Waldo, an attorney in Washington State, an active advocate for induction loops, also spoke at the convention.

Ellen Semel, a member of the Manhattan chapter of the HLAA and chair of the HLAA NYC Loop Committee, points out that looping helps only some of those with hearing impairment. It is of no use to the profoundly deaf, for instance. A person with a hearing aid but without a telecoil can access the system with headphones. The Justice Department is considering mandating induction loop systems in chain movie theaters, though nothing has come of this as yet. Semel told me that many of the movie chains are now introducing captioning devices, including eyeglasses that show captions, or handheld devices. The movie theaters, she says, are being proactive in anticipation of a federal mandate.

During all this kerfuffle over a new hearing aid and assistive listening devices that would work with both it and my implant, I realized I needed to switch to an audiologist at the Implant Center. I regretfully left Therese, though I imagine she may not have been overly sorry to see me go—my case was getting too complicated. I saw a lovely woman named Audrey, who fitted me with a great new hearing aid and all the assistive devices. Shortly after that, she moved to Washington, so now Megan is my audiologist for both hearing aid and implant.

7. *And Then You Have to Pay for It*

The relative decrease in the cost of hearing aids also takes into account inflation. "Hearing Aid Cost," April 5, 2010, on the website Healthy Hearing, gives the cost of hearing aids as ranging from $1000 to $4000. Most other sources give a range of $2000 to $6000.

The Pew Research report, "Nearly Half of American Adults Are Smartphone Users," appeared on PewInternet, March 1, 2012. *The Guardian* reported on the Gartner research under the headline "Half of UK Population Owns a Smartphone," October 31, 2011.

Change in the rulings on flexible spending accounts is discussed on Quinnscommentary.com, February 17, 2011: "PPACA changes the rules for Flexible Spending Accounts. Is fighting that change justifiable?"

Suzanne Kimball's research, published in *Hearing Journal*, March 2008, noted: "The clinical impact of this research appears to be far-reaching. First and foremost, online hearing tests can misrepresent the severity of hearing loss. That, in turn, raises doubts about the prescribed hearing aid settings derived from the online test results." The follow-up study comparing hearing aid fittings also appeared in *Hearing Journal*, March 2009.

In the six or eight months between the time I first wrote about online hearing aid sales and the time I went back to double-check the information, the offerings had changed drastically. Online retailers had toned down their sales pitches, and Amazon.com appeared to have virtually stopped selling hearing aids. Comments like those from Buckeye Hornbrook were no longer to be found.

The FDA definitions of hearing aids and personal sound amplification devices (PSAPs) can be found on the FDA website: "Guidance for Industry and FDA Staff: Regulatory Requirements for Hearing Aid Devices and Personal Sound Amplification Products," February 25, 2009.

The Census Bureau published these figures during Older Americans Month, May 2011.

8. *Cyborg: Cochlear Implants*

John Niparko's *Cochlear Implants: Principles and Practices*, cited above, comprises twenty-five chapters by various experts. Some are colleagues in Niparko's Department of Otolaryngology at Hopkins. The field of cochlear implantation is changing rapidly and some of the information may already be out-of-date. For instance, not only does the length of the time of implant surgery vary according to surgeon, but it gets shorter all the time. The time span cited, one and a half to three hours, is from "Medical and Surgical Aspects of Cochlear Implantation," by Debara L. Tucci and Thomas M. Pilkington in Niparko, page 168.

Michael Chorost describes himself this way: "Michael Chorost (pronounced like "chorus" with a *T* at the end) is a technology theorist with an unusual perspective: his body is the future. In 2001 he went completely deaf and had a computer implanted in his head to let him hear again. This transformative experience inspired his first book, *Rebuilt: My Journey Back to the Hearing World.* He wrote about how mastering his new ear, a cochlear implant, enabled him to enhance his creative potential as a human being." His description not only of the surgery but of the workings of a cochlear implant is detailed and clearly written. This description of the surgery appears on pages 33–34. The story about Graeme Clark's finding the solution to fitting an electrode array into the spiral cochlea is described on pages 36–37.

The description of the electrode array is also from the chapter in Niparko cited above, page 166.

The package insert that came with my Advanced Bionics Harmony HiResolution Bionic Ear System warns that people with implants should not be in the area where an MRI scanner is located. In the event that an MRI scan of the brain is essential (to rule out a brain tumor, for instance), the implant surgeon can temporarily remove the magnet in the imbedded receiver and thus render the scan safe.

John Oghalai and many co-authors wrote about NIRS imaging in a paper titled "Neuroimaging with Near-Infrared Spectroscopy Demonstrates Speech-evoked Activity in the Auditory Cortex of Deaf Children Following Cochlear Implantation," *Hearing Research* 270 (2010). He also talked to me about it when I visited Stanford in the spring of 2012.

"Curing Hearing Loss," by four Stanford researchers, including Stefan Heller, appeared in the *Journal of Communication Disorders*, Volume 43, Issue 4, July–August 2010.

The statistics about cochlear implants are much more reliable than statistics about hearing loss, because they do not depend on self-reporting. The numbers cited are from the NIDCD website on implants, with information provided by the FDA.

Blake Wilson and Michael Dorman's "The Design of Cochlear Implants" appears in Niparko, pages 97–98.

In 2010, Arizona made cutbacks in Medicaid that ruled out liver transplants for patients with hepatitis C, as well as lung transplants and certain heart, bone-marrow, and pancreas transplants for any Medicaid patient. It also dropped 47,000 low-income children from the Children's Health Insurance Program.

Information about brain plasticity and the age at which neurons are no longer produced comes from Ryugo and Limb, "Brain Plasticity: The Impact of the Environment on the Brain as It Relates to Hearing and Deafness." The impact of early stimulation on the auditory system is discussed on page 32, in Niparko. The quote about the lack of success in implanting prelingually deafened adults is on page 28. The quote about prelingually deafened adults eventually benefiting from implants is on page 33.

The 2007 review article on children with implants and academic achievement is interesting not only for itself but for the studies it cites in "Effects of Cochlear Implants on Children's Reading and Academic Achievement," by Marc Marschark,

Cathy Rhoten, and Megan Fabich (all at the Center for Education Research Partnerships, National Technical Institute for the Deaf), *Journal of Deaf Studies and Deaf Education*, Volume 12, Issue 3, pages 269–282.

Both *Sound and Fury* and *Sound and Fury: Six Years Later* are available on Netflix.

The discussion of the sound quality of cochlear implants appears in "Correlates of Sensorineural Hearing Loss and Their Effects on Hearing Aid Benefit and Implications for Cochlear Implantation," by Ryan M. Carpenter in Niparko, page 86.

9. Wig Tape, and That Pig Outdoors

I recommend Kisor's book to anyone who has ever tried to speech-read—and for anyone with hearing loss, for that matter. *What's That Pig Outdoors? A Memoir of Deafness*, by Henry Kisor, Hill and Wang, 1990. This quote appears on pages xv to xvi.

10. How to Be a Deaf Theater Editor, and Other Challenges of Real Life

Curious about the term "Shouts and Murmurs," I asked a *New Yorker* researcher about its origins. "Shouts and Murmurs," Jon Michaud told me, was the title of Alexander Woollcott's collection of pieces about the theater. The term "Shouts and Murmurs" refers to the technician in charge of offstage noises. Speaking of deaf theater editors—and in this case, critics—I came upon the interesting fact that Woollcott had mumps in his early twenties, which is thought to have left him impotent. Hearing loss is a very common complication of mumps. Did he have hearing loss? Woollcott was known for his quips, but not for carrying on a meaningful conversation. (Wolcott Gibbs said of Alexander Woollcott's column, which he edited: "I guess he was one of the most dreadful writers who ever existed.")

A looping system is not a "hearing aid," as the description makes clear. It works *with* a hearing aid or cochlear implant. *New York Times*, November 23, 2011.

Hearing loops are also discussed in chapter 6. Ellen Semel was very helpful in correcting my misunderstandings.

11. The Ugly Stepsisters: Tinnitus and Vertigo

Much of the information about tinnitus comes from MarkeTrak VIII: "The Prevalence of Tinnitus in the United States and the Self-Reported Efficacy of Various Treatments," by Sergei Kochkin, Richard Tyler, and Jennifer Born in *Hearing Review*, November 2011. Although estimates range from 30 to 50 million sufferers, this study put the number at 50 million: "A recent self-report survey using the 1999–2004 National Health and Nutrition Examination Surveys (NHANES) database on more than 14,000 subjects estimated that 50 million US adults reported having any tinnitus and 16 million reported frequent tinnitus in the past year."

Robert Dobie's article, "Overview: Suffering from Tinnitus," appears as chapter 1 in *Tinnitus: Theory and Management* by James Byron Snow. The comments about prior problems with depression appear on page 4. Tinnitus, Dobie remarks, "is not inherently very unpleasant; it causes suffering in large part because of the meanings that people attach to it, for example, 'It is a sign of serious disease,' 'I am going to go deaf,' 'It will get worse,' or 'I cannot control it.' "

Jerome Groopman's article appeared under the title "Medical Dispatch: That Buzzing Sound: The Mystery of Tinnitus," *The New Yorker*, February 9, 2009.

The quote from Darwin's letter appears in *The Correspondence of Charles Darwin: Volume 13, 1865*, edited by Frederick Burkhardt et al., Cambridge University Press, 2003.

That it was tinnitus that drove Van Gogh to cut off his ear (actually only part of it) is one of many diagnoses that have been offered, including acute intermittent porphyria and bipolar disorder. All were discussed in an article in the *Washington Post*: "Van Gogh's Madness: The Diagnosis Debate Lives On," by Megan Rosenfeld, November 22, 1998.

The quote from Beethoven appears in "Beethoven's Deafness and His Three Styles," *British Medical Journal*, December 20, 2011.

The Letterman-Shatner interview, March 18, 1996, can be accessed on YouTube.

Except for Will.i.am, the information about musicians with tinnitus is collected on the website The Buzz Stops Hear or other similar sites, including hearnet.com: "Celebrities and Musicians with Tinnitus." Original sources and some details are given for all.

The use of hearing aids for tinnitus is discussed in "Hearing Aid Amplification and Tinnitus: 2011 Overview," *Hearing Journal*, June 2011.

The 2010 issue of *Hearing Journal* devoted to tinnitus should be of interest to anyone who suffers from it, especially if it has been dismissed as "psychological" or of minor importance. Articles cited in the text are not included here. Robert Sweetow and Jennifer Henderson Sabes's overview of management techniques is especially useful. The pharmacological treatments of tinnitus are discussed in "A guide to pharmacologic management of target symptoms of severe tinnitus," by Linda S. Centore, *Hearing Journal*, November 2010. Other articles discuss ginkgo biloba, Ring Stop, and Quietus.

The Hopkins paper on the treatment of vertigo with dexamethasone was titled "Longitudinal Results with Intratympanic Dexamethasone in the Treatment of Ménière's Disease," by Maria Soledad Boleas-Aguirre, Frank R. Lin, Charles C. Della Santina, Lloyd B. Minor, and John P. Carey, *Otology and Neurology*, January 29, 2008. John Carey discussed this work, as well as a different paper on the use of intratympanic gentamicin for Ménière's-induced vertigo that appeared in *Audiology and Neurotology* in 2009, in an interview at Hopkins in the spring of 2011.

12. Chicks and Fish Do It. Why Can't We?

The Hearing Health Foundation's symposium, "The Promise of Cell Regeneration," was held at the New York Academy of Medicine on October 3, 2011. The occasion was the kickoff of the foundation's Hearing Restoration Project. Information about the project's funding and consortium members comes from Andrea Boidman, the executive director of the foundation. The full symposium is available at drf.org/hri, with subtitles available. The quotes from the meeting are all from a transcript of the event.

In the spring of 2012, I visited Ed Rubel at the University of Washington, where I also met with Bruce Tempel. At Stanford I met with Stefan Heller, John Oghalai, and others. Robert Jackler was also interviewed at Stanford in the spring of 2012. All the researchers quoted have read and corrected the passages about their work. Any remaining errors are mine.

Stefan Heller announced the successful attempt at regenerating hair cells in a 2010 paper in the prestigious journal *Cell*, under the title "Mechanosensitive Hair Cell-like Cells from Embryonic and Induced Pluripotent Stem Cells." The authors were Kazuo Oshima, Kunyoo Shin, Marc Diensthuber, Anthony W. Peng, Anthony J. Ricci, and Stefan Heller, all from Stanford.

The report on NAC appeared in *The ASHA Leader* under the title "A Magic Pill?" on June 14, 2005.

I also visited Jonathan Kil when I was in Seattle in the spring of 2012, at Sound Pharmaceuticals, a tidy set of offices in a suburban neighborhood with a lab in the basement. We put on paper slippers to go in and see the technicians at work and the mice in cages who are the study subjects.

Acknowledgments

I want to thank the many physicians and researchers who generously shared their work and their thinking with me, and who promptly responded when I came back time and again, asking for clarification. At Johns Hopkins, Drs. John K. Niparko, John P. Carey, Frank R. Lin, Brad May, Charles Limb, Paul Fuchs, and Elisabeth Glowatzki talked to me at length about their research, and in some cases offered elementary courses in basic otolaryngology. At Harvard, Charles Liberman walked me through the pioneering work that he and Sharon Kujawa are doing on the effects of noise on hearing. At the University of Washington, Dr. Ed Rubel and his colleagues allowed me to sit in on a freewheeling conversation about the possibilities and limitations of the search for a biological cure for hearing loss. Dr. Rubel also read and reread much of chapter 12, as did Dr. Stefan Heller at Stanford. Also at Stanford, Dr. John Oghalai let me try out his work in progress, tentatively called the cochleoscope. Dr. Robert K. Jackler, chair of the Department of Otology and Neurotology at Stanford, talked with such conviction and vision about his department's work that it was easy to see how he has attracted such a celebrated staff of researchers. (In the interest of space, I have omitted "Dr." in the text, though in most cases the researchers are both M.D.s and Ph.D.s.)

Many people with hearing loss shared their stories with me. Some are named in the book. Others wished to remain anonymous. I learned a tremendous amount about my own hearing loss from these conversations, and for the first time ever I got to know others like me. The composer and record producer Richard Einhorn was among them. His background in acoustics made him a knowledgeable reader as well as an astute observer of his own deafness. He read the manuscript in an earlier form and made many helpful suggestions.

The Cochlear Implant Center, part of the Ear Institute at the New York Eye and Ear Infirmary, sometimes seems like my second home. Dr. Ronald Hoffman, who has been my ENT for decades (and who is the only "Dr." in the text, because that's what I call him), has put up with endless anxious questions about causes and prognoses with unflappable patience. Megan Kulhmey and Elizabeth Ying have both contributed to helping me learn to hear again with the cochlear implant, nudging me to work harder when my spirits flagged. I have often felt that the entire staff at the Implant Center was watching my back, so thank you all.

For early—and in some cases repeated—readings of my proposal and manuscript, and for their tireless encouragement, my thanks to Robin Marantz Henig, Susan Engel, Dinitia Smith, Katha Pollitt, Leslie Garis, Cornelia Dean, and the many friends who listened to me think out loud. I especially want to thank Dr. Eslee Samberg, whose wisdom and insight helped me see my way out of the despair that can accompany deafness. Going deaf is a little like finding oneself in the Slough of Despond, minus the sin. In *Pilgrim's Progress*, Bunyan writes: "This miry slough is such a place as cannot be mended . . . For still as the sinner is awakened about his lost condition, there arise in his soul many fears and doubts, and discouraging apprehensions, which all of them get together, and settle in this place . . ."

My agent, James Levine, saw the promise in my proposal and over many drafts helped make this book a reality, enlisting not only the entire staff at Levine/Greenberg to read it repeatedly but also his wife, a psychologist, as well as his wife's friend, also a psychologist. My editor, Sarah Crichton, is so unfailingly enthusiastic, supportive, and wildly generous with her praise that she makes me try as hard as I can to live up to it. Dan Piepenbring, Sarah's assistant, fills in the practical blanks and is gratifyingly prompt and informative. (And he liked my title.) I was dazzled by the professionalism and thoroughness of the entire FSG staff, including my production editor, Susan Goldfarb, for arranging for deft and subtle editing. Jenny Carrow came up on a first try with a cover design that swept me off my feet with its beauty. Thanks to Jeff Seroy and his staff, including Lottchen Shivers, for getting the word out. And to Jonathan Galassi, who gathered all this talent into one place, and then let me be part of it too.

In some ways, this book was a family effort. My son, Will Menaker, transcribed many of the interviews and made many helpful comments. My daughter, Elizabeth Menaker, fact-checked several chapters and was an unfailing cheerleader. My sister, Jean, drove me all over Seattle to interviews, and my aunt Marjorie braved the traffic morass that is Boston, Cambridge, and Somerville to find researchers in the most remote places. My husband Dan's exceedingly high literary standards have made my own writing far more precise and literate than it would have been without him. And although I've been downright impossible to live with from time to time—going deaf isn't easy—he's always been there for me.

Index